HK 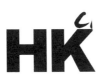 EATS

2003 Edition

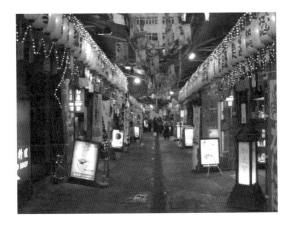

Nicole Lade

Plover Cove Limited
Hong Kong

HK Cheap Eats

ISBN 962-86732-1-1

First edition – December 2002
First published – December 2002

Published by:
Plover Cove Limited

P.O. Box 33761,
Sheung Wan,
Hong Kong.

Tel: (852) 2549 1770
Fax: (852) 8148 9818
www.plovercove.com.hk
eats@plovercove.com.hk

Front cover photograph:
Katiga Street, Hung Hom, Kowloon (Nicole Lade)

Design:
Sarah Woods
smwoods@bigfoot.com

Printed in Hong Kong

At the time of printing, all information was verified. However, the Hong Kong
restaurant scene changes frequently, so please send any corrections, additions
or other information and enquiries to eats@plovercove.com.hk.

Table of Contents

Brief Bites   215

Quick Reference Guide   221

Introduction

There's no doubt that dining in Hong Kong can appear a little daunting. Potential language barriers aside, there are about 9,500 restaurants in the territory (according to the Hong Kong Government), and Hong Kong is generally renowned as being an expensive city.

Hence the arrival of HK Cheap Eats - an easy-to-use guidebook that includes more than 250 of Hong Kong's budget dining options. Restaurants right across the territory - well known or not, covering all different cuisine types - have been included.

Comprehensive information accompanies each recommendation, such as the restaurant's contact details, business hours, whether or not it offers takeaway, and which credit cards it accepts. A Quick Reference Guide listing cuisine by location and other useful information is also included at the back of the book.

So next time you are hungry but don't want to 'break the bank', pick up this guide for some independent advice about the best value restaurants that Hong Kong has to offer.

Many thanks to the following people who have assisted in putting together this guidebook: Iris Cheung, Doris Cheung, Sarah Woods, Oliver Woods, Vikki Maver, Katrina Goli, Kylie Uebergang, Jo Oswin, Alan Wong, Mark Laming and Pete Spurrier.

Happy eating!

About the Guide

HK Cheap Eats is a comprehensive guide containing more than 250 of Hong Kong's best value restaurants. Inside the guide you will find independent restaurant recommendations and other practical information.

How the restaurants made it into HK Cheap Eats
The key criteria to make it into this guide is that the restaurant must offer most, if not all, its main meals at $60 or less each. It is then intended that once a drink and another course is added in, the total price of the dining experience would be about, or less than, $100.

About the recommendations
Each recommendation provides an independent insight into the restaurant's food, service, prices and environment. The restaurants are listed by location - firstly split into the major geographic divisions of Hong Kong Island, Kowloon, the New Territories and the Outlying Islands, and secondly by area - and then by name; the cuisine type is also easily recognized. The recommendations are accompanied by helpful information such as the restaurant's contact details, business hours, if it offers takeaway, and which credit cards it accepts, if any.

What else is in the guidebook?
The 'Tips for Budget Dining' section identifies budget dining hot spots and other hints for eating on the cheap in Hong Kong.

In the 'Brief Bites' section, some budget dining restaurants are also listed without the addition of comprehensive information.

The 'Quick Reference Guide' at the rear of the book lists restaurants by cuisine and location, making it easy to search for a restaurant in the location and with the cuisine type of your choice. There are also other useful listings highlighting restaurants that are vegetarian only, provide a non-smoking section, have extended hours (including those that are open very early (7am or before), very late (1am or after) and 24 hours), and a list of favourites - restaurants that come highly recommended for their price, food, service, location or a combination of each. At the rear of this section, you'll also find a listing of all the branches of the restaurants reviewed.

Other notes
All monetary amounts referred to are in Hong Kong Dollars.

The spelling of the same dishes sometimes varies between restaurant recommendations. In each case, a standardized approach has not been taken and, where known, the individual restaurant's own spelling of the dish has been used.

It is common practice for restaurants to add a '10% Service Charge' on top of the bill for the meal. The prices quoted in this guidebook are exclusive of this charge. This extra amount generally goes directly to the restaurant (and not to the waiters or waitresses) so, if you believe that the service provided was worthy of a tip, it is best to give extra money on top of the bill.

Tips for Budget Dining

Budget dining hot spots

While cheap restaurants can be found all over Hong Kong, there are some areas where budget dining venues have congregated. These are:

- 'Rat Alley', Wing Wah Lane, Lan Kwai Fong

- Chungking Mansions, Nathan Road, Tsim Sha Tsui

- Hau Fook Street, Tsim Sha Tsui

- 'Katiga Street', Sung Kit Street, Hung Hom

- Temple Street, Jordan

See the relevant sections in the guidebook for more information on each of these hot spots, as well as for restaurants located in these areas.

Food halls and food markets

Food halls are generally located in the basement or on the ground floor of large shopping centres and provide a decent place to sit, usually a non-smoking environment, and a range of cuisines to choose from.

Food markets - serving local style fare in a hawker style environment - are located inside the former Urban Council services building in each district, usually on the floor above the wet market.

Tea Sets

The ubiquitous tea set - a combination of a meal and a drink, but at a much discounted rate - is a Hong Kong icon.

Mostly starting in the mid-afternoon, but sometimes also at a more lunch-appropriate hour, and finishing before dinner, 'tea sets' are offered by many restaurants.

Go local

Pack the phrase book and try out one of the thousands of local eateries, known in Cantonese as 'dai pai dongs'. The food is the cheapest around and you'll make new friends with the other patrons who you'll undoubtedly have to share a table with.

Veggies and squid

Hong Kong is a meat lover's paradise but things aren't all bad for vegetarians - prices for vegetarian dishes are usually the cheapest on the menu, sometimes $20 less than the meat prices. Note though that 'vegetables' in a cheaper Chinese-style restaurant are almost always only one variety - choi sum.

If you love seafood, the cheapest option (often by a long way) is squid. Luckily, it comes in a range of cooking styles so as to avoid 'squid boredom'.

Use this guide!

All the hard work has been done... all you have to do is eat!

See inside for more than 250 of Hong Kong's best value restaurants across a range of locations and cuisine types.

Hong Kong Island

Home to a large expatriate population and the prime business centre, Hong Kong Island offers the most numerous and diverse range of restaurants in the territory.

Economical eateries are located all over the island including on the south side – at Stanley, Shek O and Repulse Bay, in the east – at Quarry Bay, North Point and Taikoo Shing, and then on the north side in Wanchai, Happy Valley, Causeway Bay, Admiralty and The Peak, and into the Central area – including Lan Kwai Fong, SOHO (South of Hollywood Road), the International Finance Centre (IFC), and the Mid-Levels.

A key budget eating hot spot is Wing Wah Lane in Lan Kwai Fong, Central, otherwise known as Rat Alley. Good-natured touts will proposition you to eat at their restaurants and you can choose from a range of cuisines including Chinese, Vietnamese, Thai, Malaysian and Indian. It is one of only a few places on Hong Kong Island where patrons can sit outside, in a fun and balmy atmosphere.

EAT

Shop 008, LG1,
Pacific Place,
88 Queensway,
Admiralty

2868 3235

Hours:
M to Sa: 8am-9.30pm
Su & PH: 10am-9.30pm

Takeaway: Yes
Credit Cards: V,MC,AE

EAT, located on the Lower Ground Floor at Pacific
Place, bills itself as 'not just another sandwich
shop'. The decor is very 1950s American diner
style - with lightweight stainless steel everywhere
- and it sits perched on a couple of small raised
levels.

The food is fast and also diner style - that is, you
fill up a tray as you move along the food display
counter to the cashier. Along the way, you'll find
salads ($20 to $55), cold and hot sandwiches
(average $40), sushi (around $40), pizza and
pasta, and hot dogs (all for $36). Then there are
dessert and cakes ($10 to $25), snacks like ice-
cream and crisps, and juices and other beverages
to choose from.

EAT offers a good range of decently-priced food,
in a fast and healthy-enough style, to satisfy most
hungry shoppers and moviegoers.

Great Food Hall

Hours:
10am-10pm daily

LG1, The Mall,
Pacific Place II,
88 Queensway,
Admiralty

Admiralty

Takeaway: Yes
Credit Cards: V,MC,AE

2918 9986

Pardon the pun, but the Great Food Hall is a great place to eat a great meal. Located at the bottom of Pacific Place, it offers a range of cuisine all cooked fresh to order.

In typical food hall style, you'll find Korean, Thai, Chinese, Italian and Western style food, as well as desserts and drinks all available under the one roof. But, in a non-typical food hall set-up, the food is prepared by Great itself and not various vendors. There's plenty to choose from and the prices are reasonable. Pasta, for example, spinach linguini with tomato, eggplant, garlic and basil, is a treat at prices ranging from $42 to $58; and noodles, for example, canton dumplings with noodles in soup, are cheap at $22. There's also a carvery serving roast meat and all the trimmings for $50.

If you are in a hurry, pre-made sandwiches, salads and juices are also available from inside the supermarket area.

Piazza Italian/Cafe

Unit 009, Level LG1,
The Mall, Pacific Place II,
Queensway,
Admiralty

2918 0630

Hours:
M to F & Su: 10am-10pm
Sa: 9am-10pm

Takeaway: Yes
Credit Cards: V,MC,AE

Located in the Pacific Place basement, opposite the Great Food Hall and within the Great supermarket, is the Piazza restaurant.

Designed as a cosmopolitan café, Piazza serves Italian and café style meals at all times of the day. Breakfast is served until 11am, and then everything else is offered until the 9pm closing time. There are stylish sandwiches and salads available for $42 to $52, while the speciality pizzas start at $65. There are also desserts (tiramisu is $28), ice-cream, cakes and pastries, and a range of beverages to suit your sweet or thirst needs.

The Piazza is a nice place to relax with a coffee, or something more substantial, without the 'food-hall' feel.

Food Hall   **The Food Fare**

Hours:
10am-9.30pm daily

1/F, Pacific Place,
88 Queensway,
Admiralty

Admiralty

Takeaway: Yes
Credit Cards: None

2801 4197

Pacific Place (known as P.P. to the locals) is a modern, stylish shopping centre and its food hall, The Food Fare, is testimony to this. Imbued with brown tones with interesting lighting and trendy seating, this place even makes two of its chain outlets - KFC and Café De Coral - look good.

But you don't have to stop there because you'll find Singaporean food at the Noodle Place at around $28; an average priced Thai curry or noodle dish at Patong Thai for $30; and steamed rice meals at the Chinese outlet - Super BBQ - for $23.

Don't despair if you've spent all your money on your P.P. shopping spree - all you need is some loose change to enjoy the range of delights at the Food Fare, in a setting that'll make you feel rich.

CitySuper Cooked Deli   Food Hall

Basement,
Times Square,
1 Matheson Street,
Causeway Bay

2506 2888

Hours:
M to Sa: 8.30am-10pm
Su & PH: 10.30am-10pm

Takeaway: Yes
Credit Cards: None

CitySuper's Cooked Deli, connected to the CitySuper supermarket in the basement of Times Square, offers a choice of Korean, Japanese, Chinese, Indian, Thai and Western style cuisine with a centralized cashier and seating space.

As an example of some of the meals available: the Fusion Deli has toasties for $23, sandwiches for $28, and herb chicken cream sauce with penne for $35; Yoshimoto Chaya offers a teriyaki chicken steak set for $45; and Curry in a Hurry has a vegetarian executive set for $45.

With inexpensive food to suit all tastes, the Cooked Deli is a great place to grab a bite, in a non-smoking environment, when taking a break from shopping.

See the Branches section for details of the Tsim Sha Tsui Cooked Deli (also reviewed).

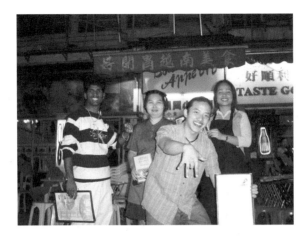

▲ Good-natured touts in Lan Kwai Fong (PHOTO: Nicole Lade)
▼ One of Lan Kwai Fong's roti makers (PHOTO: Nicole Lade)

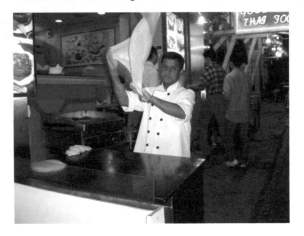

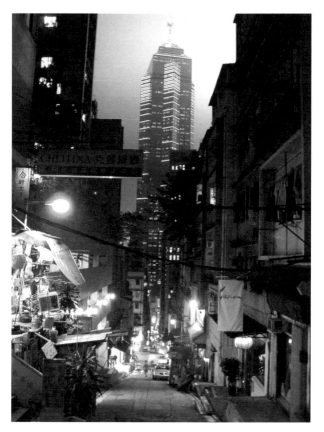

▲ Peel Street - it bisects SOHO's Elgin and Staunton Streets, descends through a wet market, and then disappears into a network of dai pai dongs in the shadow of The Centre. (PHOTO: Sarah Woods)

Chinese　　　**East Lake Seafood**

Hours:
10am-12am daily

Takeaway: Yes
Credit Cards: V,MC,AE,D

2504 3311

Step into the East Lake restaurant in the mornings
or afternoons and you step into the world of
Cantonese dim sum.

This large and noisy restaurant is very popular -
especially before 12.45pm (11.30am on Satur-
days and Sundays) or after 2pm when the dim
sum is offered at discounted rates (starting at a
cheap $8.80, usually for three pieces). All the
dim sum favourites are here - including cha siu
bau (roasted pork buns), shrimp dumplings and
taro cakes - either served to the nicely laid table
by polite waiters or eaten buffet style. During
lunch and dinner times, the prices for other meals
are also quite reasonable - for example, rice and
noodle dishes start at $22, and three beers are
$10.

The East Lake is a good place to practise your
Cantonese but an English menu will materialise if
you're having trouble with the nine tones.

Go Go Café

11 Caroline Hill Road,
Causeway Bay

Hours:
M to Sa: 12pm-11pm
Su: Closed

Takeaway: No
Credit Cards: None

2881 5598

There's one word to describe Go Go Café - cosy. The food and atmosphere are 'homely' and the generous portions are served on nice crockery.

As an example of the food and prices: salads, such as the warm chicken avocado salad, are generally $55; sandwiches range from $42 to $45; and pasta, for example, the spicy sausage spiral pasta with tomato sauce, and rice dishes are all around $55. The few main courses, such as steak, are in the $60 price range. Organic and fruit tea and drinks form a large part of the menu and there are also homemade desserts, including tiramisu for $27, to tempt you.

The Go Go Café is not bad for a relaxed and comfortable reminder of home dining experiences.

Vietnamese   **Green Cottage**

Hours:
11am-11pm daily

G/F, 32 Cannon Street,
Causeway Bay

Takeaway: Yes
Credit Cards: V,MC

2832 2863

The Green Cottage Vietnamese Restaurant has the 'same boss, different kitchen' as Yin Ping (also reviewed) and was the first restaurant of the two to open. The menus and prices of each restaurant are similar, but the Green Cottage's menu is a little more traditional.

Vegetable lovers are well catered for at Green Cottage - the fried vegetable dishes are $38 and include fried sugar pea shoots with garlic, and fried lettuce with bean curd. The signature Vietnamese dish - cold noodles - is $27; and the rice dishes, like Vietnamese fried rice, range from $27 to $48. The restaurant's recommended dishes, including the curry eel, beef or duck ($50), are all served with bread, thanks to Vietnam's French legacy.

Like Yin Ping, the dining style is fast, and overall the food and service is reasonable.

Heart Café   Cafe

Shop A, G/F,   **Hours:**
10 Pak Sha Road,   M to Sa: 10:30am-10:30pm
Causeway Bay   Su: 2:30pm-10:30pm

                                          Takeaway: Yes
2882 7884   **Credit Cards:** V,MC

The Heart Café doesn't offer too much in the way
of menu choice but it's a quick, cheap and clean
place for a bite.

Most of the items on the menu are tea and coffee
but there are some café style meals to choose
from. There are sandwiches, for example, roast
beef and vegetable, available for around $30;
salads, for example, a Caesar, for a maximum of
$25, and a range of set meals (lunch, sandwich,
soup and salad) that are around $40. The cakes
in the window look inviting - for example, lemon
or mango cheesecakes are $28. Don't be
surprised if the food tastes and looks Chinese
style, even though it has Western names.

The Heart Café is okay for a pit-stop while taking
a break from the Causeway Bay draw-card -
shopping.

Indonesian   **Indonesian Restaurant**

Hours:
11:30am-10:30pm daily

Takeaway: Yes
Credit Cards: V

28 Leighton Road,
Causeway Bay

2577 9981

The Indonesian Restaurant is an institution in Causeway Bay and, in fact, in Hong Kong. The restaurant has been open since 1968 and has a loyal following of patrons including Hong Kongers and diners who are originally from Indonesia.

While the décor still represents the '60s, the Indonesian food is the authentic kind that withstands time. For example, gado gado is tasty at $48; daging Bali (beef with chili sauce) is hot at $58; and the satays are juicy at $40. You can also take home Indonesian goods, like kopi (coffee), which are displayed for sale in the restaurant's window.

Large groups are well catered for at the Indonesian Restaurant, which makes dining with friends, and sharing the great food, even more of a treat.

Mini Paris

Vietnamese

23 Canal Road West,
Causeway Bay

Hours:
11am-11:30pm daily

2591 4015

Takeaway: Yes
Credit Cards: V,MC,AE

As you walk into the Mini Paris Vietnamese Restaurant (see the Branches section for other locations), you feel like you've entered a hut. With chairs made of cane and walls lined with bamboo, the atmosphere is calming (compared to the Canal Road madness out front), and the staff are eager to please.

The standard Vietnamese dishes are pretty cheap (interestingly, you have to pay $1 extra on Saturdays and holidays), for example, the pho averages $20 and fried noodles and bun are around $21. More exotic and expensive dishes are also on the menu, including fried frogs legs with butter for $53; chicken wings fried with lemongrass for $34; and vermicelli dishes for around $40.

The use of fresh herbs certainly brings out the flavours and, overall, the food is worth trying at this popular restaurant.

Vietnamese   **Perfume River**

Hours: 89 Percival Street,
11am-11pm daily   **Causeway Bay**

Takeaway: Yes
Credit Cards: V,MC,AE   2576 2240

With 227 items presented in an indexed menu,
one good thing about the Perfume River
Vietnamese Restaurant is that there's plenty to
choose from.

Most dishes start from $28. As an example: the
pho (soup with noodles) ranges from $26 to $36;
the cold vermicelli with shrimp or Vietnamese
salami and chicken are both $32; and the beef
brisket curry and rice is $45.

While the food is generally tasty and the
restaurant is conveniently located (right on the
Happy Valley tram line and just near Times
Square), the food is a bit overpriced compared to
other Vietnamese restaurants in the area, and the
absence of windows tends to create a
claustrophobic atmosphere.

Thai-Jade

Thai

G/F, No. 50,
Leighton Road,
Causeway Bay

2808 0734

Hours:
11:30am-2am daily

Takeaway: Yes
Credit Cards: V,MC

The Thai-Jade restaurant is nothing to look at from the outside, but inside the menu is comprehensive and the prices are relatively cheap.

Fried prawns with cashew nuts and chili is $50; chicken, fish, beef, duck and vegetable curries are all $40; and vegetables and noodle and rice dishes are up to $40. The tom yum kung is recommended ($40 for a small) and so too the not-so-typical desserts (around $20).

With two restaurants in Causeway Bay (also nearby at G/F, No. 10, Matheson Street, 2808 0462), these two down-to-earth eateries are a good find for an authentic and decently priced meal.

Indonesian

Warung Malang

Hours:
10am-10pm daily

2/F, Flat B-2,
Dragon Rise Building,
9-11 Pennington Street,
Causeway Bay

Takeaway: Yes
Credit Cards: None

2915 7859

The Indonesian Consulate is located in Causeway Bay and consequently a 'little Indonesia' has cropped up in its vicinity.

Warung Malang is a small restaurant-in-a-room that offers home-cooked Indonesian meals, fast food style, to mostly Indonesian expatriates. 'Others' are welcome though and you will be greeted with true-blue Indonesian hospitality, even before you walk in the door. The tasty meals are all around $25 to $30, including the favourites like gado gado and nasi campur.

Warung Malang is also a small centre to buy Indonesian food and music products, and is a nice place to feel part of a community atmosphere, especially on a Sunday when it's the amahs' day off.

Yin Ping

Vietnamese

G/F, 24 Cannon Street,
Causeway Bay

Hours:
11am-11:30pm daily

2832 9038

Takeaway: Yes
Credit Cards: None

The first thing you notice when you enter Yin Ping is that there is no music playing - there's just a gentle hum from happy diners. The second thing you become aware of is that an attentive staff member has shuffled you into a seat, most likely at a table shared with others, and a pen and paper has been placed in front of you for you to write your own order. And there's plenty to choose from.

Most rice dishes are $29, including the Vietnamese fried sausage with rice; hotpots are $52; and the cold noodles are all around $27. There's a feast of snacks and the cold pork and shrimp rolls are light and tasty at $23. The meal portions are generous and the staff are extremely attentive.

After enjoying your meal, and before you know it, your table has already been wiped clean and another hungry diner is waiting to take your seat.

Café   **? Coffee**

Hours: Shop 5B, Cheung Fai
M to F: 8:30am-8pm   Building, 45-47
Sa: 10am-8pm   Cochrane Street,
Su: 12pm-6pm   **Central**
Takeaway: Yes
Credit Cards: None   2581 2128

Even though ? Coffee's address quotes a busy
walking thoroughfare, it's actually situated in a
small alleyway just off the main drag, meaning it's
a nice and relatively quiet place to visit.

As its name suggests, ? Coffee's menu offers a
long list of coffees, and most are available hot or
iced and small or medium sized. A mocha is $19
for small size and hot, or a hazelnut macchiato is
$26 for medium size and iced. Where there's
coffee, there's also tea and, in ? Coffee's case,
there's also sandwiches, bagels, salads, toasties,
soup and cakes. Sandwiches range from $24 to
$35; bagels are $12 to $20; and the salads and
wide range of toasties are mostly $24. Breakfast,
lunch and tea sets are also available.

The shop itself is quite small but overall the food
and coffee on offer are good value, especially for
its Central location.

3 Piggyz Grill   Burgers

76 Wellington Street,
Central

2118 1383

Hours:
M to Th: 12pm-10pm
F to Sa: 12pm-4am
Su: Closed
Takeaway: Yes
Credit Cards: None

The adage 'cheap and cheerful' is a perfect description of the 3 Piggyz Grill - a small eatery that offers value-for-money gourmet hot dogs, cheese steaks and burgers, all served quickly and in a friendly manner.

The '100% natural' sausages, for example, the all beef, foot-long frankfurter called the 'Top Dog', or the self-explanatory 'lemon chicken', go for a cheap $22. There are tasty cheese steaks including the 'philly' for $40, or $45 for the 'deluxe' and the 'classic'. Then there's three beef burgers for $30 to $35; side orders, like French fries, that range from $8 to $20; and plenty of soft drinks and relatively cheap beer.

With a set meal available that includes sausage, cheese steak or burger plus a side dish plus drink for $15 more than the meat only price, this is a great place for a quick, cheap and tasty meal.

Lebanese

Beyrouth Café

Hours:
12pm-11:30pm daily

Takeaway: Yes
Credit Cards: V,MC,AE,D

Shop A, G/F,
Lyndhurst Building,
No. 39 Lyndhurst Terrace,
Central

2854 1872

Conveniently located, Beyrouth Café offers fast and delicious Lebanese cuisine that is as close as you are going to get to a typical U.K. High Street kebab shop.

The kebabs get good reviews from all who eat them - the chicken kebab (shawarma), for $45, has even been described as 'the best kebab in Hong Kong'. The meat is cut directly from the kebab spike then fried in front of you, before being tossed into the light and not too thin pita bread. The salads and sauces that are then added, for example, the mint garlic sauce, are also deliciously fresh. As well as kebabs (which all go for around $45) you can choose from other Lebanese delights like hommos and baba ghannouj dips for $38, or tabbouleh for $45.

You can sit at bench seats but the café is really more a takeaway joint. Beyrouth is a must-visit place for kebab fans.

Café Le Bleu   Café

G/F, Union Commercial
Building,
12 Lyndhurst Terrace,
Central

2543 8962

Hours:
7am-8pm daily

Takeaway: Yes
Credit Cards: None

Café Le Bleu is a small coffee and sandwich shop
that is relatively modern with maritime (and
washed-out blue) themed décor. It seems to
have built up a dedicated following and it's
common to see loyal patrons drop in to say
'hello', show off their new haircut, or just take a
rest.

All the standard Western style café fare is
available, including sandwiches from $25 to $35,
salads for $35, fresh juice for $20, and also
yoghurt, muffins and desserts. There is an array
of coffee on the menu, including café latte for
$28, and tea, for example earl grey, for $18.

Cafe Le Bleu is a nice place to sit and relax, read
the paper or just chat, in a very central location.

Café   **Dailybread Café**

Hours:
M to Sa: 7am-10pm
Su: 7:30am-7:30pm

Takeaway: Yes
Credit Cards: None

Shop No. 118,
Yip Fung Building,
No. 14–18 D'Aguilar St.,
Central

Central

2868 6013

The Dailybread Café occupies a prime location just at the base at Lan Kwai Fong, making people-watching an added bonus to eating here.

As the name suggests, the Dailybread Café offers bread, salads, sandwiches and drinks, either as set meals or as make-your-own orders. Breakfast is served from 7.30am to 10.30am, with a choice of three sets, including the 'full breakfast' for $32. For lunch, there are a number of sets available, ranging from $27 to $40, which generally include a sandwich and salad, with various ingredients, and a drink.

The salad and sandwich fillings are very 'Hong Kong standard' (meaning ham, egg, crab meat and so on), but the prices and the two-storey view make a visit here worthwhile.

See the Branches section for details of other locations.

Hot Dog   Hot dogs

27-29 Hollywood Rd.,   **Hours:**
Central   Open 24 hours

                             Takeaway: Yes
2543 3555   **Credit Cards:** None

One good thing about Hot Dog is that it's open 24
hours.

Another good thing is that it's cheap. The classic
hot dog is $20; the 100% beef hot dog is $22; and
the most expensive item on the menu is the
jumbo (ten inch) sausage for $30. You can also
pay for extras like coleslaw, onions and
sauerkraut.

Unfortunately, the hot dogs are 'mediocre',
although they do taste okay at 4am after a big
night out.

A redeeming quality is that Hot Dog also sells
alcohol and cigarettes - a plus in the early hours
when there is no 7 Eleven close by.

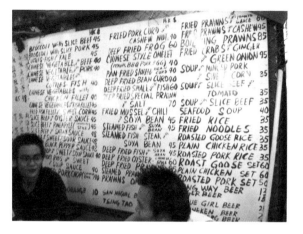

▲ Menu on the wall in Temple Street (PHOTO: Nicole Lade)
▼ Temple Street fare (PHOTO: Nicole Lade)

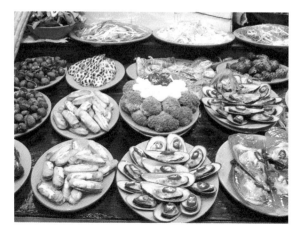

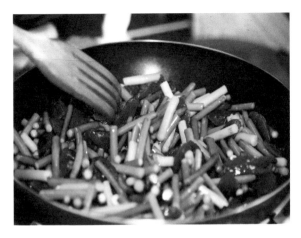

▲ Ubiquitous green vegetables (PHOTO: Kylie Uebergang)
▼ Busy fresh juice bar in Central (PHOTO:Sarah Woods)

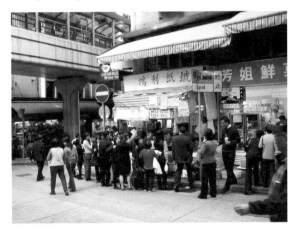

Cyber Café

IT Fans Cyber Café

Hours:
Open 24 hours

Takeaway: Yes
Credit Cards: None

Unit A & B, G/F,
Cockloft Man On
Commercial Building,
No. 12–13 Jubilee St.,
Central
2542 1868

Located right in the heart of Central, this two-floor Cyber Café is a good find.

The price to use the computers is reasonable ($18 per hour for non-members), the atmosphere is 'professional', and there's also a range of food available to munch on while gaming or surfing. The food is not gourmet but it's what you'd expect from this type of place. You can get noodles from $18; sandwiches and snacks from $8; fish and chips for $20; and rice or spaghetti dishes from $35. Malaysian curries are a speciality; you can order them from $32 to $35, or as part of a set that not only includes a drink but also one hour free Internet and online game usage.

So if you're up for 24 hours worth of cyber activities, and you're hungry, then venture no further than IT Fans.

Koshary Cafe   Egyptian

G/F, Shop A,
112-114 Wellington St.,
Central

2544 3886

Hours:
M to Th: 10am-11pm
F to Sa: 10am-1am
Su: 11am-11pm
Takeaway: Yes
Credit Cards: V,MC

The Koshary Café, the cheaper version of next door's sister restaurant, Habibi, offers a fine sampling of Egyptian cuisine that is unique in Hong Kong.

The café has two menus - Café by Day and Café by Night. For the budget-minded, it's recommended that you visit during the day when the cheaper menu is available. As an example of the tasty, value-for-money food from the daytime menu: hot and cold mezze platters range up to $38; Egyptian style sandwiches (including shawarmas) are around $40; and heartier selections include Egyptian mussaka for $40 or $50 (vegetarian or lamb respectively). The balawa bil ishta or baklava ($25) is highly recommended; it's moist and will melt in your mouth.

The food and service at Koshary Café are above average, and if you're lucky you may be treated to a belly dancing show.

Mak's Noodles

Hours:
11am–8pm daily

G/F, 77 Wellington St.,
Central

Takeaway: Yes
Credit Cards: None

2854 3810

Opposite Tsim Chai Kee noodle shop (also reviewed), Mak's Noodles offers tasty and cheap Chinese fare and a larger menu than its neighbour.

The cheery chef in the window will welcome you into the light and clean, old and local style restaurant. The usual dishes are on the menu including wontons for $23 and noodles and briskets for $35. The beef brisket is particularly tasty - the beef tastes very beefy, more like it does in a Western style beef stew than in a Chinese style brisket.

Venture into Mak's for a taste of Hong Kong that is very much enjoyed by locals and expatriates alike.

They also have a branch in Causeway Bay - see the Branches section for details.

Noodle Box   Asian

G/F, Shop 3,   **Hours:**
30-32 Wyndham Street,   M to Sa: 12pm-10:30pm
Central   Su: Closed

                                            Takeaway: Yes
2536 0571   **Credit Cards:** None

If you want to sample some decent noodles (not only Chinese style), Noodle Box is a relatively quiet, cosy and trendy place to visit.

Usually their noodles are $45, but between 3pm and 6pm Monday to Friday it's 'Happy Hour' and all noodles go for $28. The noodles come in good portions, with tasty no-MSG flavours, and include Hokkien noodles with roast duck, and vegetarian laksa with mushrooms, tofu and Shanghai bak choy in a spicy coconut broth. There are also daily specials and side orders available, like Chinese greens for $20.

Noodle Box is an inviting place to eat at if you are a solo diner, and the high stools and bar top tables make people-watching on the street outside attractive too.

Tsim Chai Kee Noodles

Hours:
10am–9pm daily

Shop B, G/F,
Jade Centre,
98 Wellington Street,
Central

Takeaway: Yes
Credit Cards: None

2850 6471

Tsim Chai Kee is definitely worth a visit. Not only is it unique and locally famous but it is also extremely cheap.

Why is it unique? There are only three items on the menu - king prawn, fish ball or sliced beef dumpling noodles. And how cheap is cheap? Each of the items is only $10! Sure, you sit on shared tables and the décor is nothing flash, but who cares when you get excellent food for a bargain price? A dish of choi sum can be ordered extra for $5 and soft drinks are also $5.

If you are on a budget or you want to experience a locally famous gastronomical institution, look no further than Tsim Chai Kee Noodle shop.

Tsui Wah Restaurant Chinese

G-2/F,
15-19 Wellington St.,
Central

2525 6338

Hours:
6am-4am daily

Takeaway: Yes
Credit Cards: None

Tsui Wah Restaurant is locally famous. It's huge (it has three floors for dining), it's open early and late and offers fast food in a noisy and crowded environment.

All the usual Chinese style fare is on offer. Noodles in every form, including Japanese udon, macaroni and spaghetti, are available, as well as rice (Chinese and Western style), curry and fried dishes. And there are salads, sandwiches, drinks and, of course, set meals to choose from. Standard noodle dishes go for an average of $25, sets are $30 to $40, and most other meals are in the $40 range.

There's nothing too pretentious about the place and the food is nothing special. But the locals love it, and keep going back, so check it out for a cultural experience if nothing else.

Zhong Guo Song

Hours:
M to Th: 11am–10.30pm
Sa & Su: 11am–10.30pm
F: 11am–11pm
Takeaway: Yes
Credit Cards: V,MC

G/F, 6 Wo On Lane,
Central

Central

2810 4040

Zhong Guo Song boasts homestyle cooking - with no MSG - and over 100 menu items to choose from.

It also offers a discount scheme, which is good news for budget diners. For example, if you dine in and finish eating before 12.45pm, you receive a 20% discount. The food is not too badly priced even if you decide to eat during the peak, non-discount times. For example, fried noodle with choi sum, mushroom and chicken will set you back $38; braised chicken Hainan style is $48; and steamed squid in preserved shrimp sauce is also $48.

Zhong Guo Song is a good option for a wholesome - and potentially discounted - taste of China.

Eating Plus Asian

1009, 1/F, International
Finance Centre,
1 Harbour View St.,
Central

2868 0599

Hours:
M to Sa: 7:30am-10:30pm
Su: 7:30am-9:30pm

Takeaway: Yes
Credit Cards: V,MC,AE,D

Eating Plus is hip and huge. The restaurant décor is all stainless steel and minimalist furniture and the area is large, open, clean and spacious. It even has a mission statement printed inside the menu - 'healthy eating means healthy living'.

Vegetables, noodles, pasta, rice, risotto and fresh juices are the main fare here. For example, the vegetarian rice paper rolls are $27, and the chicken teriyaki broth noodles, the fettuccini with mushroom and broccoli, and the pan-fried risotto with Japanese pumpkin are all $58. There's a separate juice bar which pumps out glasses full of health for $18 or less.

If you're feeling hip and healthy, or if you want to, then Eating Plus is the place for you. If not, then just come for the feeling of open space (as long as it's not too busy) not often found in Hong Kong.

Bagels

Manhattan Bagels

Hours:
M to F: 7:30am-7:30pm
Sa: 9am-5pm
Su & PH: Closed
Takeaway: Yes
Credit Cards: None

2028, 2/F, International
Finance Centre,
1 Harbour View St.,
Central

2525 6080

Expatriate North American bagel experts rate Manhattan Bagels as one of, if not 'the', best bagel places in town.

There are lots of different varieties of 'emotionally gratifying' bagels, speciality cream cheeses, meat, vegetable and cheese fillings, and pre-defined bagels to choose from, as well as salads, fruit, muffins, croissants and beverages. Most of the bagel 'sandwiches' - for example, the typically named '7th avenue', which includes a choice of bagel and grilled chicken, avocado, cottage cheese and lettuce - are $40, or you can custom-build your own for around the same price.

There's no seating in the shop but there are seats available just outside. For a great taste of North America, with fresh and different fillings, look no further than Manhattan Bagels.

Nine to Five

International

2016, 2/F, International
Finance Centre,
1 Harbour View St.,
Central

2295 0100

Hours:
M to Sa: 7am-6pm
Su: 8am-5pm

Takeaway: Yes
Credit Cards: None

This cheap restaurant offers all the basics and a
few others at a quality consistent with the price.
Don't let that put you off though, especially if you
are after one of the cheapest meals around.

There are sandwiches that range in price up to
$29; soup for $9; pies for $10; hotdogs as
'snacks' for $17; fried eggs for breakfast for $17.
50; and instant noodle, vermicelli and macaroni
dishes for up to $19. The most expensive item on
the menu is a set Chinese meal for $34; and
there are Western 'combo' meals (Chinese style
'Western' though) for $33.

For the cheapest meal at the IFC with business
hours longer than its name suggests, look for Nine
to Five.

They also have another branch in Central - see
the Branches section for details.

Cafe

Pret A Manger

Hours:
M to F: 7:30am-6:30pm
Sa: 8:30am-6:30pm
Su: Closed
Takeaway: Yes
Credit Cards: None

1003B-5, 1/F,
International Finance
Centre,
1 Harbour View St.,
Central
2520 0445

For those who haven't experienced Pret A Manger in another part of the world, the 'café' offers a range of healthy and eco-friendly sandwiches, juices, soups, cakes and cappuccinos in a standardised, semi-industrial, smoke-free setting.

Everything is cooked, made or juiced fresh on the day. The sandwiches are made with brown bread, and you can choose from the Pret salad, which includes hummus, red onions, red and yellow peppers and salad, for $25. The tuna is dolphin-safe, of course, and you can purchase a tuna and mayo baguette for $26. The juices, including carrot, coconut and blueberry combinations, are all around $22, and soups, for example minestrone, are around $15.

To experience what's on offer at Pret A Manger before it becomes ubiquitous in Hong Kong, venture to the IFC (or see the Branches section for other Central locations) for a dose of fresh, healthy, original food at okay prices.

Ramas Coffee

Cafe

2020, 2/F, International
Finance Centre,
1 Harbour View St.,
Central

2295 1788

Hours:
M to F: 9am-11pm
Sa & Su: 9am-7pm

Takeaway: Yes
Credit Cards: V,MC,D

Ramas is not a bad place to hang out at while waiting to catch the train to the airport, or even for lunch or dinner. There's a large screen with music videos playing, magazines to read, and the Internet to surf.

They bill themselves as a coffee place but there's a decent sized food menu to choose from. Pasta dishes go for around $60; noodles are in the $50 to $60 range, including a pork laksa for $50; salads are generally $60; or, for an Asian snack, lemongrass chicken wings are $42. There are also sandwiches, hotdogs, pizzas, burgers and even tacos.

Yes, the prices are at the higher end of the cheap scale but, for this, the food quality is decent.

Bar / Food   **Zentro**

Hours:
M to Th: 12pm-1am
F & Sa: 12pm-12am
Su: Closed
Takeaway: Yes
Credit Cards: V,MC,D,AE

2022, 2/F, International
Finance Centre,
1 Harbour View St.,
Central

2899 2221

If you're seeing someone off to the airport (but perhaps not actually going to the airport) or looking for a bar with food in a central and convenient location, then Zentro is the pick of the bunch at the IFC.

Seating is at the bar, at high tables near the entrance (ideal for wheeling airport trolleys up to) or at standard tables. The bar/eatery offers a range of tasty food but the snack menu - served from 3pm to 10pm - is the best for economical eating. There are about ten menu items, including homemade bruschetta for $40, deep fried cheddar with pommery mustard dip for $50, and Thai styled fish cakes flavoured with lemongrass, also for $50.

The portions are quite large and will do for either a generous snack or as a meal if you're not too hungry.

Bon Appetit   Vietnamese

14B, G/F,
Wing Wah Lane,
D'Aguilar Street,
Central

2525 3553

Hours:
10am-12am daily

Takeaway: Yes
Credit Cards: None

A narrow restaurant with not much street
presence, Bon Appetit is sometimes overlooked in
Rat Alley. But if it's cheap and good Vietnamese
food you're after, then try this small eatery.

Everything is priced at $33 or less, and includes
an array of Vietnamese dishes including rice,
noodles, vermicelli (cold and dry), baguettes,
desserts and drinks. The vegetarian bun (cold
vermicelli) for $24 is light and tasty, so too the
Vietnamese noodle roll for $22. There's a menu
with pictures to help you decide what to eat.

Look for the restaurant with yellow seats, tucked
in between Club 64 and the Taste Good Thai
restaurant, and you won't go wrong.

Asian   **Café de lankwai fong**

Hours: 20 – 22 D'Aguilar Street,
10am-2:30am daily   **Central**

Takeaway: Yes
Credit Cards: V,MC,D   2525 6628

A relative newcomer to the Lan Kwai Fong
gastronomical scene, Café de lankwai fong offers
different Asian style meals.

Even though from the outside the restaurant looks
like a typical, albeit new, Chinese restaurant, the
menu covers Chinese, Thai, Malaysian,
Indonesian and Japanese cuisines. As an
example of the fare: the Thai red curry with
chicken and vegetable is $48; Japanese fried rice
with assorted pickles is $42; and the Indonesian
nasi goreng is $52.

The prices are quite decent for this area, and the
availability of different cuisines makes a visit here
even more tempting.

Co Co Curry House   Malaysian

G/F, 8 Wing Wah Lane,
Central

Hours:
11am-3pm
& 6pm-12.30am daily

Takeaway: Yes

2523 6911

Credit Cards: V,MC

Many a diner has watched in awe the antics of the artistic roti man at the Co Co Curry House. Not only does he prepare the roti at his outside workbench in a way you've never seen before, he also performs tricks when serving tea - right at your table.

And the food is worth coming for too. The curry laksa in soup is pretty hot at $40 and the beef madras is hotter at $50. Nasi goreng is $45 and, for vegetarians, the mixed vegetable curry comes with a two-chili hot rating for $40. You must try the roti that you watch being flipped and pounded; both the signature Co Co roti and the banana roti are $30.

You can watch the roti man from most of the other Rat Alley restaurants, but for a full view and some good food at the same time, you might as well join the other impressed diners here.

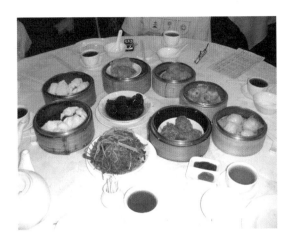

▲ Dim sum – a local favourite (PHOTO: Iris Cheung)
▼ Shop and eat 'til you drop in Stanley (PHOTO: Iris Cheung)

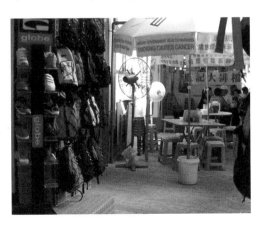

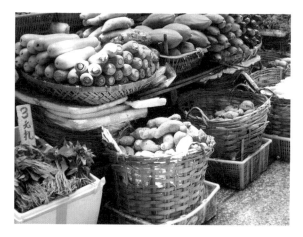

▲ Vegetables in season at the market (PHOTO: Nicole Lade)
▼ Noodle guys (PHOTO: Sarah Woods)

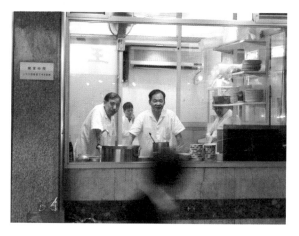

Thai   **Good Luck Thai**

Hours: G/F, 13 Wing Wah Lane,
M to Sa: 11am-2am   **Central**
Su: 4pm-12am

Takeaway: Yes
Credit Cards: V,MC   2877 2971

You are guaranteed a good meal at the Good Luck
Thai Food Restaurant. The friendly staff will
always find you a seat somewhere in the crowded
outdoor seating.

There's an extensive menu to choose from,
including a large vegetarian section; for example,
sautéed seasonal vegetables is $35, or for meat
lovers, the sautéed pork with chili and pepper is
$40. The sautéed seasonal vegetables and squid
($48) is always tasty, and so too is the fresh squid
in red curry paste ($45).

With probably the most outdoor seating, and good
food at reasonable prices, this place is a good
choice to soak up the lively, down-to-earth Rat
Alley atmosphere.

India Curry Club   Indian

Shop M & L, 3/F,
10 Wing Wah Lane,
Central

2523 2203

Hours:
11:30am-3pm
& 5:30pm-10:30pm daily

Takeaway: Yes
Credit Cards: V,MC,D

If you feel like Indian food but you're not sure how to get to this restaurant, head up 'Rat Alley' and Lan Kwai Fong's very own Elvis look-alike will lead you in the right direction. Three floors up, you enter a mixed atmosphere - typical Indian cum Rat Alley - as you enter the India Curry Club.

The food is definitely worth coming here for. The fish vindaloo ($60) is 'spot on' - that is, it has a bit of a kick to it - and the fish is tastily fresh. For vegetarians, the navarathan korma ($45) leaves your taste-buds feeling happy and you healthy and full. There are the usual Indian tandoori, chicken, lamb, seafood, breads and rice dishes here - mostly priced in the $40 to $50 range - but no beef dishes.

Come here for some of the best, and most reasonably priced, Indian food on the Hong Kong side of the harbour.

Sandwiches / Pizzas

La Baguette

Hours:
M to Th: 10am-1am
F & Sa: 10am-4am
Su: 11am-9pm
Takeaway: Yes
Credit Cards: V,MC

G/F, 18 Lan Kwai Fong,
Central

2868 3716

La Baguette doesn't only offer baguettes or French food, as its name might suggest. In fact, it offers more Italian style cuisine - salads, pastas, grills, desserts, sandwiches and pizzas - right in the heart of Lan Kwai Fong.

Most of the main meal dishes start at $70 but the sandwiches and pizzas are cheaper and worthy of a mention. The sandwiches and toasties come with a choice of breads and one, two or three tasty fillings, like avocado and brie, or cheddar, tuna and pickle, and are priced from $38. Then there are the pizzas that can be topped with most of the same ingredients as the sandwiches and toasties. Prices start at $55 for a small, $75 for a double, and $98 for a large - the latter two sizes could easily be shared for a cheaper meal.

La Baguette has a great location, with bench seating for street-viewing, and an interesting array of fillings and toppings that the Western palate will certainly appreciate.

Midnight Express   International

No. 3, G/F,   **Hours:**
Lan Kwai Fong,   10am-3.30 am daily
Central

2525 5010   **Takeaway:** Yes
                          Credit Cards: None

If it's 4am - and you're hungry and looking for a
quick, cheap snack, in the centre of all bar
happenings - then this is the place to come.

There are a few diverse items to choose from:
kebabs are all around $55 for a large or $40 for a
small; curries are $30; moussaka with salad is
$40; and the beef Cornish pasty is also $40.

Beer is more reasonably priced here than at other
places close by, so it's possible to enjoy a cheap
beer while standing in the street eating your
gyros.

The general consensus however is that Midnight
Express is a place to visit for food only after
you've had (or are having) a few drinks. They
also have a branch in Wanchai at G/F, 88 Lockhart
Road, 2520 6117.

Thai

Taste Good Thai

Hours:
M to Sa: 11am-1am
Su: 6pm-12am

No. 16 Wing Wah Lane,
Central

Takeaway: Yes
Credit Cards: V,MC,D,AE

2523 9543

The Taste Good Thai Food restaurant certainly lives up to its name. Just on the right at the top of the lane when you walk up to Rat Alley, the restaurant offers seating inside or outside and a large selection of always-tasty Thai food.

Recommended dishes include the spicy and sour squid salad ($48); the spring rolls ($38); and the red curries ($48 or $52 for pork/beef/chicken or squid respectively). If those items don't suit your fancy, then there is a range of salad, vegetable, rice, noodle, and Thai and curry delights to do so.

Not much more needs to be said about this restaurant than 'it's good' and definitely worth a visit.

Chicken on the Run

Shop A, LG/F,
No. 1 Prince's Terrace,
Central

Hours:
11:30am-9:30pm daily

2537 8285

Takeaway: Yes
Credit Cards: V,MC

If you like chicken 'to go', then Chicken on the Run is for you. It's clean and bright and conveniently located alongside the escalator.

As the name suggests, the menu offers all things chicken, to take away. This includes whole chickens and wings cooked in different ways and with different seasonings. The meals available include a range of salads and chicken pieces for $25 to $60, depending on the size. There are also rice and chicken dishes that go for around $40.

There's some bench seating and, interestingly, a small section selling a range of olive oils inside the outlet. And don't be concerned about Hong Kong chicken and the bird flu; Chicken on the Run uses chicken from overseas countries such as Australia.

Russian   **Czarina Express**

Hours:
11.15am–9.30pm daily

Shop B, G/F,
Kam Fung Mansion,
59-61 Bonham Road,
Central

Takeaway: Yes
Credit Cards: None

2104 9988

Czarina Express is the fast-food version of the original and more expensive Russian eatery, Czarina Restaurant.

Even though you might have to wait a few minutes for the food, it's worth waiting for. The bortsch is $26 and is as good as the sister restaurant's version. Set meals are around $40 to $45; the curry vegetable is $30; and the chicken or prawn salad is $35. There are salads, main courses and canapes that are on offer for groups of eight to ten people to take away - these work out to be around $50 per head, depending on the meal and group size. A-la-carte rice or spaghetti dishes are also available for take away, including the garoupa with sweetcorn sauce for $40.

To sit in or take away, look for the green sliding doors and the diner style eatery, and you've found the Czarina Express.

Lee's Patisserie

Patisserie

G/F, 49 Lyttelton Road,
Central

Hours:
M: Closed
Tu to Su: 11am-9pm

Takeaway: Yes

2559 9765

Credit Cards: None

Lee's Patisserie is a small eatery with a cosy, neighbourhood feel. Firstly, it's a patisserie with mouth-watering cakes, tarts, pies and quiches available to enjoy there or to order for takeaway or delivery. Secondly, it offers a small menu for eating on the spot.

Salads and sandwiches, including the farmer's salad for $38, and South East Asian noodles, rice and spaghetti dishes, including the lamb curry and spaghetti bolognaise, both for $48, are available. Seating is mostly inside but there's a small table outdoors.

Enjoy Lee's Patisserie for its relaxed, out-of-the-way atmosphere and for its homestyle cooking.

Malaysian
Malaya Restaurant

Hours:
11am–11pm daily

Shop 1D, G/F,
37-47 Bonham Road,
Central

Takeaway: Yes
Credit Cards: None

2548 4980

The Malaya Restaurant is an interesting meal option if you are in the area. The menu is quite diverse but Malaysian style food dominates.

For the 'best in Malaysian food', there are curry and rice dishes ranging from $38 to $60, half a dozen satays for $35, sambals for around $45, laksas for an average $40, and rice and noodle dishes for $38. Then there's a large range of international meals including soup, salad, steak, rice, noodles, spaghetti, sandwiches and cakes, with just about everything available for $60 or less.

The popular restaurant is reasonably sized, the spices are authentic-tasting, and the staff are attentive. Come here for a taste of Malaysia or to experience some samples of other countries' cuisines.

Mini Kitchen

Mid Levels, Central

G/F, 17A Bonham Road,
Central

Hours:
11am-10pm daily

Takeaway: Yes
Credit Cards: None

2915 2531

Mini Kitchen is a mix of Chinese and Western styles. This pertains not only to the décor - on the outside, it has a weatherboard façade with quaint door-lamps, and inside, tables are covered with red-chequered tablecloths - but also to the food.

There are cheap, more Chinese style meals on offer for $20 to $26, including baked garoupa with rice for $22; or slightly more expensive, a-la-carte Chinese-Western style meals ranging up to $60. For example, a grilled lamb chop dish is $60, or a beef, chicken or ox-tongue curry is $38. Soup, salad, sandwiches, rice and spaghetti meals are also available, including a club sandwich for $42.

If the not-so-tempting food display out the front of the restaurant doesn't put you off, then venture into the Mini Kitchen for its own version of how East meets West.

Monterey Chicken

Hours:
12pm–10pm daily

Shop 1, G/F,
31-37 Mosque Street,
Central

Takeaway: Yes
Credit Cards: V,MC

2526 6896

A takeaway outlet only, Monterey Chicken caters for individual and group eaters alike, and is proud to claim that it uses 'only imported poultry and all natural herbs and spices'.

Anything chicken is available including whole chickens, cooked using their 'original' or their signature 'Thai style' recipes for $65; or the half chicken combo, which includes a choice of two side dishes (for example, mashed potato or mixed vegetables) for $45. Then there are wings and drumsticks for $5 and $15 respectively. If you're not into chicken, there are also some non-poultry dishes available, including BBQ ribs for $40; hot and cold sandwiches, ranging from $15 for a jumbo hot dog to $25 for a grilled beef burger; and salads from $20 to $30.

'Super value meals' also cater for groups of four or eight and work out to be good value at around $40 a head.

V-Twin Cafe American

G/F, 30 Bonham Road,
Central

Hours:
Tu: Closed
M to Su: 11am-11pm

Takeaway: Yes
2186 7812   **Credit Cards:** None

V-Twin is an industrial-looking but cosy restaurant. Its menu is fun to read, not only because of the tasty-sounding American style meals on offer but also because the menu developer obviously considers him or herself something of a comedian (as well as a motorbike enthusiast).

For example, there are snacks to 'try for a happy tummy'. This includes onion rings for $22 which, according to the humorous menu writer, you are allowed to consider part of your daily vegetable intake. Burgers go for $38, pasta is $45, and the super hot dogs, which come with fries, range from $32 to $36. Breakfast lovers will be happy to hear that there's a fry-up available all day for $46.

With magazines to read and a variety of meal options V-Twin, as the menu says, is 'a cool place to hang out and fuel up'.

Deli / Mexican **Archie B's / Taco Loco**

Hours:
12pm-12am daily

LG/F,
7-9 Staunton Street,
Central

Takeaway: Yes
Credit Cards: None

2522 1262

As relative newcomers to the SOHO dining scene,
these two restaurants receive good reviews all
round. Archie B's is a delicatessen that offers
New York style speciality sandwiches as well as
deli sandwiches, salads and meats, whereas Taco
Loco provides Mexican favourites like tacos,
burritos and tortillas.

On the deli side, most of the specially named
sandwiches (NYPD Blue, for instance) are $60 or
more and could easily be shared for economical
eating. Salads are available for $50 and deli
favourites like hot dogs are even less. At Taco
Loco, the tacos and burritos start at $12 and $28
respectively.

Just as good, the restaurants are located in a
convenient position right on the escalator, just
down from Staunton Street, and offer high-table
outside seating in the small lane adjacent. Drop
in to try two of the latest places that everyone's
been talking about in this part of town.

Gourmet Kitchen   International

G/F,
34B2 Staunton Street,
Central

2522 2162

Hours:
Su to Th: 12pm–11pm
F & Sa: 12pm–12am

Takeaway: Yes
Credit Cards: None

The Gourmet Kitchen offers international cuisines to take away or for delivery only so don't come here expecting a sit-down meal.

There's a huge list of Western, Chinese, Italian and Mexican dishes to choose from, and skeptics may wonder how one kitchen can produce decent food from such a huge, mixed cuisine menu. Well, you'll have to try for yourself and you won't be disappointed. You can choose Chinese food like fried rice or curry starting at $48; Western food like Cajun chicken Caesar salad for $50; Mexican nachos also for $50; and the Italian spaghetti carbonara for $60. Kids' meals, side dishes, desserts, drinks and set meals are also available.

The Gourmet Kitchen is not a bad choice, especially if you are eating with diners of mixed palates and you have somewhere else to eat.

Crepes   **Le Rendez-vous**

Hours: G/F, 5 Staunton Street,
10am-11:30pm daily   **Central**

Takeaway: Yes
Credit Cards: None   2905 1808

Le Rendez-vous is first and foremost a French creperie.

Savoury crepes, with interesting names like 'the marine' (salmon, spinach and egg) and 'the brunch' (egg, bacon, mushroom and tomato), are available for $45. Then there are sweet crepes and waffles like 'the French kiss' (vanilla ice-cream, chocolate and almonds) and the classic 'lemon sugar' (butter, sugar and lemon) that range from $20 to $45. Or you can even create your own for $25 plus $8 per extra topping. Baguettes, salads, buckwheat rolls and toasted panini, with a range of fillings, are also available for around $35 to $40.

You can dine in or take away - the eatery is tiny so the latter is not a bad option. Enjoy Le Rendez-vous for its unique fare, which you won't find elsewhere in Hong Kong, and for its relatively reasonable prices.

Southern Restaurant   Chinese

G/F, 49 Elgin Street,
Central

Hours:
11am-2:30pm
& 5pm–12am daily

2841 8878

Takeaway: Yes
Credit Cards: None

If you come here during the non-business hours
of 2.30pm to 5pm, don't be surprised to see the
chef snoozing on tables pushed together inside.
But if you come during opening hours, you'll be
treated to a feast of Chinese food served in this
traditional looking restaurant.

The chef's special is chicken and scallop congee,
which goes for $20. Fried rice and noodle dishes
average around $32, and hotpots are generally
$50. Fish dishes, including the fried sliced squid
with broccoli, are a little more expensive but peak
at $60.

The Southern Restaurant is a good addition to this
mostly Western (or non-Chinese) dining strip but
just choose your visiting hours with care.

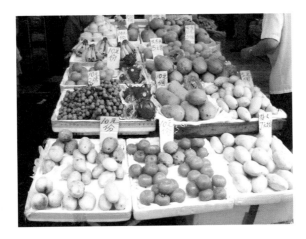

▲ Fruit in the market (PHOTO: Nicole Lade)
▼ Tasty barbequed meats (PHOTO: Nicole Lade)

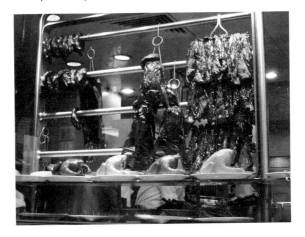

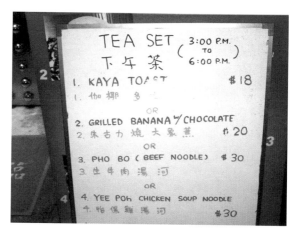

TEA SET (3:00 P.M.
TO
6:00 P.M.)

下午茶

1. KAYA TOAST   #18
1. 伽 梛 多 士

OR

2. GRILLED BANANA ⁄ CHOCOLATE
2. 朱 古 力 燒 大 象 蕉   # 20

OR

3. PHO BO (BEEF NOODLE)   # 30
3. 生 牛 肉 湯 河

OR

4. YEE POh CHICKEN SOUP NOODLE
4. 怡 保 雞 湯 河   # 30

▲   Tea time – a good value time to eat (PHOTO: Nicole Lade)
▼   Fish hanging out to dry (PHOTO: Kylie Uebergang)

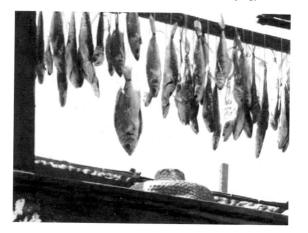

Bakery / Bagels   **The SOHO Bakery**

Hours:
8am-8:45pm daily

G/F, Shop B1 and B2,
41 Elgin Street,
Central

Takeaway: Yes
Credit Cards: V,MC,D,AE

2810 7111

The SOHO Bakery and The Bagel Factory sell their
delicious breads, cakes and patisseries on a
wholesale basis across Hong Kong, but they also
offer a taste of their fine wares at this small retail
outlet.

On The Bagel Factory side of the shop, you can
choose from a range of different bagel 'flavours',
including blueberry, cinnamon and wholewheat as
well as cream toppings, and an array of salads
that are available for, on average, $15 per 100g.
There are also pita bread wraps, including chicken
pita, for $30. On the SOHO Bakery side, you can
choose such delights as chocolate fudge, brioche,
croissants and baguettes.

All this and more can be eaten in with a drink, or
taken away, or even catered for you if you are
holding a party or junk trip.

The Corner Shop   International

43 Staunton Street,
Central

2543 2632

Hours:
M: 5pm-1am
Tu to Su: 10am-1am

Takeaway: Yes
Credit Cards: None

Located on the same corner site as the former Kantipur, The Corner Shop has retained the laid-back, open (no walls) and bench-seating style made popular by the previous restaurant. But, moving up in the world, The Corner Shop is more modern and has an expanded menu.

You'll still find Nepalese cuisine and fish and chips but now there are Italian favourites like ravioli, lasagne and linguine, as well as chicken any-way-you-like (marinated or roasted and whole, half or quarter). Prices are cheap - all dishes are $60 or less and most go for around $40. There are also sandwiches for $25 and desserts averaging $35.

You can eat 'in' at The Corner Shop and watch (and listen to) the world go by, or eat out taking advantage of their free delivery service. Either way, you won't be disappointed.

Thai   **Tom Yum's**

Hours: G/F, 36 Elgin Street,
12pm-3pm   **Central**
& 6pm-11pm daily

Takeaway: Yes
Credit Cards: V,MC,AE   2810 7318

Tom Yum's is a popular restaurant that offers Thai
food in a small and cosy environment. The food
is spicy and good, albeit at the higher end of the
cheap scale.

Rice and noodle dishes, including pad Thai and
Thai style fried rice, start at $58, and so too do
the meat dishes, including the minced pork stir-
fried with chili and basil leaves. Vegetable dishes
are a little cheaper, priced from $48 to $58,
including the tasty vegetables in peanut sauce.

Tom Yum's is conveniently located and is a great
place to visit for intimate dining.

2Rooms

Cafe

G/F, 8 Ming Fat Street,
Happy Valley

2838 2959

Hours:
M: Closed
Tu to Sa: 3pm-1am
Su: 12pm-12am
Takeaway: Yes
Credit Cards: None

2Rooms offers something a little different in Happy Valley - it's a small café style restaurant with cosy, 'cushionful' seating that has one 'room' open to the street and another 'room' located towards the rear of the restaurant.

There's not a lot to choose from on the menu - there are starters, salads and soup (for example, minestrone for $28) and the main meal is the special of the day (ranging from $48 to $80 depending on the meal and the day). Drinks are big - referring not only to the large number to choose from but also to the fact that they are generally served in small carafes (for example, the homemade lemonade is $35). For a cheapish meal, you need to pick the right day, or stick to the somewhat limited menu.

Overall though, 2Rooms is unique in Happy Valley and is not a bad place to relax in.

Billy Joe Restaurant

Hours:
7am-10pm daily

G/F, 11 Sing Woo Road,
Happy Valley

Takeaway: Yes
Credit Cards: None

2827 0811

Billy Joe's is one of those restaurants that you might notice but possibly pass by without a second glance. From the outside, it exudes the possibility of bad Chinese style Western cuisine with a fast-food feel. But on the inside, a gweilo-friendly manager, who greets his obviously loyal customers by name, will warmly welcome you.

The set meals are great value - the food is decent and the price is unbeatable. For example, for $60 you can get bortsch soup and garlic bread, followed by grilled baby lamb, rice and vegetables (albeit canned), with mint sauce served on the side, then a dessert such as fruit salad, plus tea and coffee. Great value! Other meals available include sandwiches, toast, curries and rice and spaghetti dishes, just to name a few.

There's no service charge either which means that your wallet as well as your stomach will be pleased after a visit here.

Cafe Very Good Chinese

G/F, 49-49A Sing Woo
Road,
Happy Valley

2838 3318

Hours:
7am-2am daily

Takeaway: Yes
Credit Cards: None

From the outside and peering in, Café Very Good
looks like a standard, although relatively modern,
diner-style Chinese restaurant. Inside however,
there are non-standard high-backed yellow seats
and booths, a high-tech computer ordering
system, and tasty food that is cooked with
fragrant herbs and spices.

Everything is cheap and pretty much falls into the
price range of $23 (for congee) to $32 (for noodle
dishes). Even cheaper are sandwiches - up to
$16, and rice noodle rolls starting at $13. The
fresh fish slice in soup is very tasty at $25 and,
when ordered as a takeaway, comes with the
broth in a drink container separate to the rice
noodle and fish (topped with lemongrass), and
with sachets of chili sauce to add, to make the
dish to your own taste at home.

Don't be put off by the non-English signage, Café
Very Good lives up to its name. They also have
an outlet in Central - see the Branches section for
details.

Vietnamese   **Dong Khoi**

'No MSG' boasts the sign out the front of this
Vietnamese restaurant that opens onto one of
Happy Valley's small side streets. The décor is
simple and multi-coloured - from the A4 and
postcard sized menus to the walls and to the
rattan tablemats.

The restaurant has potential but, in general, the
food and service are just okay. 'Starters' have
been known to turn up as 'enders', the food can
taste quite salty, and there's not too much to
choose from in the way of vegetarian food.
Having said that, the tenderloin beef cubes that
come with red rice ($55) are nice and tender, and
the lemongrass wings noodle in soup dish ($32) is
no-MSG-tasty with the lemongrass subtly infused
in the wings. You can also choose snacks like
spring rolls (with lettuce for rolling and dipping)
for $26, or rice and noodle dishes including a
curry beef brisket for around $40.

The iced lime juice for $18 is highly
recommended.

King's Palace

4G/F, 22 Sing Woo Road,
Happy Valley

Hours:
11:30am-12:30am daily

Takeaway: Yes
2838 4444 | **Credit Cards:** V,MC,D

The King's Palace Congee and Noodle Bar (see the Branches section for other locations) is a small, modern restaurant serving local fare.

Everything about this place is stylish - from the décor, to the Chinese and English magazines available for reading while eating, to the company-branded plastic bags used for takeaway orders.

The menu is substantial and offers tasty and traditional local meals, including congee for $35 to $38; roasted meats with rice or noodles (also around the same price range); and other snacks, for example, the King's recommended fresh pig's liver and ginger soup for $20, or the also recommended roasted eel in honey sauce at $60.

If it's local food you're after, in relatively salubrious surroundings, then you can't pass up King's.

Lotus Garden

Hours:
11am-2:30am daily

G/F, 51A & 61 Sing Woo
Road,
Happy Valley

Takeaway: Yes
Credit Cards: None

2891 5569 / 2832 9931

There are two Lotus Garden restaurants just a few
doors away from each other on Sing Woo Road,
Happy Valley's main artery.

The Lotus Garden at No. 51 is a restaurant that
offers all the usual congee, noodle and rice
dishes. While the service does not get good
reviews, the prices and food are reasonable -
noodles in soup are $30, 'noodles in dish' are
around $40 (add $5 extra for e-fu noodles), and
rice dishes are $55.

Up the road at No. 61, you'll find a feast of
desserts in a small, traditional, Chinese style
restaurant with the same name. The mango
pudding is tasty at $18, so too the mixed beans
soup for the same price. Deep boiled soup,
herbal jelly, sago and other puddings and
desserts are on offer, with some on display in the
front window, to top off your Lotus Garden dining
experience.

Mini Thai Corn

Shop A3, 67 Sing Woo Road,
Happy Valley

2838 6567

Hours:
11am-11pm daily

Takeaway: Yes
Credit Cards: V,MC

Be warned: this place has some very 'hot' food and this is not a reference to its temperature or level of 'hipness'. There are a couple of bench seats to sit at to eat one of the many dishes and set-meals, for example the (almost inedible to the sensitive palate) tom yum soup, for only $12. You can choose Thai fried rice with various toppings for around $30; or Thai fried vermicelli/noodle - for example, pat Thai - for around $33.

There's an innovative ordering system whereby you build your own meal by firstly choosing your own sauce (broth); then your noodle or rice noodle (for $5); and finally, items such as veg-etables or fish slices for $5 each, or $6 for items such as squid or chicken wings with lemongrass.

Thai speciality foods are also available at the Thai store attached to the restaurant, just around the corner.

Hours:
M to Sa: 12pm-12:30am
Su: 11:30am-12:30am

Takeaway: Yes
Credit Cards: None

G/F, 12 Ming Fat Street,
Happy Valley

2893 3336

Happy Valley

The Moon House Dim Sum restaurant is billed as a place to see famous people dining. If that's not your hobby, then it's still a good place to go for some tasty food at reasonable prices.

The restaurant is quite small and the dining atmosphere is intimate (meaning that you sit very close to fellow diners). For $58, you can choose from the seasonal specialities menu, including smoked Chinese sausage with rice in casserole, or for $49 you can select from an array of noodles or rice dishes, including Singapore style fried vermicelli. Congee is $30, desserts are around $16, and there are soup, snacks and, of course, dim sum to choose from as well.

Another word of advice: it's worth making a booking before coming here, especially on the weekend.

Moon House   Chinese / Desserts

G/F, 35 Wong Nai Chung
Road,
Happy Valley

2891 2591

Hours:
12pm-12am daily

Takeaway: Yes
Credit Cards: None

As its name suggests, the good things about this
restaurant are the desserts.

The mango pudding and red bean in coconut, for
example, taste superb and cost around $17.

The bad things are that the restaurant is small,
crowded, has slow service and just average non-
dessert food. Unfortunately, the vegetarian udon
noodles, for $33, fall into this latter category.

If you come here during a busy time, then you'll
most likely have to wait, standing up, outside the
door.

Nevertheless, a visit to sample the delicious
desserts is recommended. Just try and visit
during a non-peak time.

They also have a branch in Causeway Bay - see
the Branches section for details.

Hours:
9am-11:30pm daily

G/F, 19 Wong Nai
Chung Road,
Happy Valley

Takeaway: Yes
Credit Cards: None

2574 9537

The Motor Restaurant is easily missed even
though it is located in a very busy part of Happy
Valley - right opposite the tram terminal. Not so
impressive from the outside, this restaurant offers
a sedate atmosphere inside that is enjoyed mostly
by families seeking a quiet place for a meal out.

The meals are huge and there's plenty on offer.
The menu is split into Malaysian, French and
Chinese specialities but how the dishes were
placed under each heading is anyone's guess.
Most meals are in the $40 to $60+ range. In the
Malaysian section, you'll find curries, sambals,
laksas and (Vietnamese) noodles; in the French
section, you'll find soups, spaghetti, rice and egg
dishes; and under the Chinese section, there are
fried rice and noodles, udon and congee and
more.

The staff are attentive and the food is not bad. A
good place to come with the family or for a quiet
night out.

Island Place Food Hall

Basement, Island Place,
500 King's Road,
North Point

Hours:
M to F: 12pm-8pm
Sa & Su: 12pm-9pm

Takeaway: Yes
Credit Cards: None

Located in the basement of Island Place, this food hall does not offer the salubrious surroundings, range or quality of food as the other food halls recommended in this guide.

What it does offer though is cheap, down-to-earth food, served in a clean environment, all under the one roof. There are ten outlets offering mainly Chinese (northern and southern), Japanese and Korean cuisine. Everything is $30 or less, including a Korean BBQ combo set for $28 at Lee Jo Express, and fried udon with eel for $30 at the Japanese outlet.

The food hall is very popular, especially at lunchtime, so don't be surprised if you have to share a table.

Cafe

Java Mama

Hours:
M to F: 7am-7pm
Sa & Su: 9am-4pm

Takeaway: Yes
Credit Cards: V,MC,D,AE

Harbour Plaza Hotel,
665 King's Road,
North Point

2185 2088

Located on the ground floor of the Harbour Plaza
Hotel (North Point), on the edge of their car park,
Java Mama is a coffee shop offering café style
fare to hotel guests and the public alike. If you
can't handle ingesting the car fumes while sitting
among the plastic green hedges, there is a small
amount of seating inside.

Java Mama specialises in coffee and offers a few
brews, including a regular sized café latte for $17.
Java Mama offers a nice range of food too. There
are pastries, doughnuts and muffins available, for
an average of $13. Sandwiches go for $34,
prepared with your choice of fillings and bread;
fresh juices start at $19; salads go for around
$22; sweets, like tiramisu, are $14, and pre-made
meals like spaghetti bolognaise are also available.

The staff are friendly and there are English papers
to read, making this Western style café not a bad
find in this predominantly Chinese part of town.

Aji Ichi Ban

Japanese

Shop 1B, G/F,
Hon Way Mansion,
11 Hoi Kwong Street,
Quarry Bay

2565 8136

Hours:
11am-11pm daily

Takeaway: Yes
Credit Cards: V, MC,AE,D

If you want sushi or other Japanese fare, then Aji Ichi Ban is really the only choice in this area. The restaurant is sushi-bar style and, like the other eateries close by (and in this guide), it can get busy at lunchtime.

A sushi roll is around $18 or there are special lunch sets offering, for example, assorted sushi, udon and tea or coffee for $65. The noodles range in price from $35 to $59 and ramens are generally all around $35. There are also more substantial curry and rice dishes available for around $59 and $50 respectively.

While the food is not the best Japanese on offer in the territory - you are recommended to stay clear of the eels ('dry and full of bones') - the prices are okay. Look out for the special offers, like 20% off if you leave before 1pm, that help make this place worth a visit.

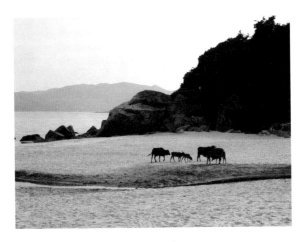

▲ Restaurant view - Cheung Sha (PHOTO: Sarah Woods)
▼ A taste of India, Chungking Mansions (PHOTO: Alan Wong)

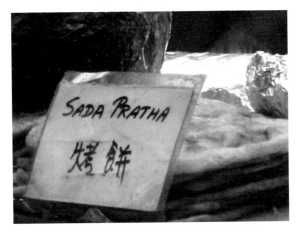

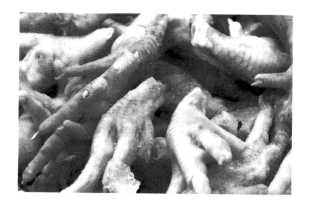

▲ Ever-popular chicken feet (PHOTO: Kylie Uebergang)
▼ Outside eating is possible year-round (PHOTO: Nicole Lade)

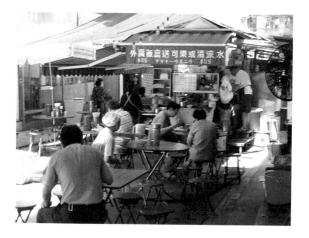

Cafe   **Crossroads Coffee**

Hours: 18 Hoi Kwong Street,
M to F: 7.30am-9.30pm   **Quarry Bay**
Sa: 7.30am-6pm
Su: Closed
Takeaway: Yes
Credit Cards: None   2565 6897

Crossroads Coffee, as the name suggests, is a
popular, modern and clean restaurant that offers
a range of coffee (and food) primarily to a
lunchtime clientele. You can choose from the
traditional coffee types including café latte,
cappuccino and iced coffee, or go for the
'nouveau' strawberry latte or cookie monster (a
creation with Oreo biscuits).

For a coffee shop, there's a fair range of food
including dishes for breakfast, lunch, teatime and
dinner, snacks and desserts, sandwiches, soups
and salads. For lunch, you can have tuna salad
with pasta for $45; for dinner, baked baby
chicken for $55; and sandwiches are all $28 (with
a choice of filling and bread).

The general feeling is that the coffee is good, the
food is average and the service is okay. So come
if you're feeling thirsty and not too hungry.

Jubal

Shop 10, G/F,
Ka Wing Building,
4-6 Hoi Wan Street,
Quarry Bay

2880 9339

Hours:
11am-6.30pm daily

Takeaway: Yes
Credit Cards: V,MC

Jubal is a relatively new kid on the block in the area and bills itself as offering 'new cuisines'. At the time of publishing, they had not been open long and were still waiting for a liquor licence.

They also didn't have a permanent menu, choosing instead to provide different dishes each day to ascertain which are popular. The menu is small, with four dishes only, ranging in price from $39 to $58. As an example of the kind of fare and prices that are (possibly) on offer: pasta of the day is $39; the hot sandwich set is $39 (and could include barbecue pork cutlet and grilled pineapple on a bun with crispy potato chips and garden salad); and the business set lunch is $58 (and might be pan-seared sea bass with coconut rice, honey bean and pineapple emulsion).

The food is above average for the area, prices are reasonable and the atmosphere is pleasant.

Cafe   **Mix**

Hours: Shop 14A, G/F,
M to Sa: 7am-8pm   Hoi Kwong Court,
Su: 9am-6pm   13-15 Hoi Kwong Street,
                                               Quarry Bay

Takeaway: Yes
Credit Cards: V,MC   2562 7313

Mix is a groovy and hip little café that offers
wraps (exotic fillings wrapped in pita bread),
salads, sandwiches and a range of smoothies for
the health, taste and scene conscious.

If you're not sure what to order, then sample the
taste-tester generally on offer at the door. The
wraps are really tasty and different to other
offerings in the area but, be quick, the speciality-
of-the-day wrap often sells out early. Classic
wraps include Cajun chicken and fajita mixicana
(salsa and sour cream) for $32 for a half and $42
for a whole. In the sandwiches area, smoked
turkey with cranberry sauce is $34 and the vegie
pesto is $36. Smoothies come in a range of fruit
combinations also with exotic names - the Stress
Buster is $36 and the Spunkey Monkey is $28 or
$32 depending on the size.

If you can't make it to the Mix in this area, then
you'll be pleased to know they also have outlets in
Central (see the Branches section for details).

Mother India   Indian

Shop No. 1,
Hoi Kwong Shopping
Centre,
13-15 Hoi Kwong Street,
Quarry Bay
2880 5334

Hours:
11.30am-2:30pm
& 6pm-10.30pm daily

Takeaway: Yes
Credit Cards: V,MC,AE,D

Some people might be surprised to find that a
good Indian restaurant exists in this part of town.
Located at the end of an inside alleyway, Mother
India serves 'the best south and north Indian
food'.

Your mouth will be watering as you smell the
spices emanating from the kitchen while reading
the very informative menu. The prices are quite
standard for the area and are reasonable for the
quality of the food. Chicken tikka is $55; rogan
josh is $60; and the vegetarian shashlik is $50.
Kashmir pullao (rice) is $42 and the naan is $10.

The restaurant is really just an oversized room,
which makes for attentive service. If you don't
work in the area then this restaurant is one that is
worth travelling out of your way for.

Cafe

Q Takeaway

Hours:
M to Sa: 11am-12am
Su: 5pm-1am

Rear of Café Einstein,
33 Tong Chong Street,
Quarry Bay

Takeaway: Yes
Credit Cards: None

2960 0994

The Q Takeaway, just near Sprouts (see review overleaf), is a good place to come for a taste of gourmet style salads similar to what is available in Western countries. There's no seating inside - which is just a small serving area - but plenty outside.

The price of the salads differs depending on the size required. For example, you can choose Caesar salad, smoked salmon nicoise and Thai beef for around $38 for a small or $48 for a large. Sandwiches are also available for $38 and there is a selection of hot foods on offer, like lasagne, that tends to change every few days.

The service is nothing to speak about, and the salads could be considered relatively expensive, but it's not a bad place to come for a reminder of food from home.

Sprouts Cafe

G/F, 23 Hoi Wan Street,
Quarry Bay

2856 9448

Hours:
M to F: 8am-9pm
Sa: 8am-3:30pm
Su: Closed
Takeaway: Yes
Credit Cards: None

Sprouts is a popular, and not too fancy, café and sandwich shop. Located on a corner, it has outside seating and a down-to-earth menu.

The sandwiches and salads are the main offerings, all coming with a feast of good fillings including alfalfa, tomato, lettuce, green pepper, onions, a choice of sauces and dressings and, for the sandwiches, a choice of breads. The brie and avocado salad or sandwich is $40, the smoked salmon is $48 and the curry chicken is $28. You can also get MSG-free homemade soup for $24, pizzas for $34 and pies for $38.

There is nothing more or less to the café than that described above, so visit if that's exactly what you're after.

Thai Cafe

Hours:
10.30am-3pm
& 5.30pm-10.30pm daily

Takeaway: Yes
Credit Cards: V,D

G/F, 7 Hoi Kwong
Street,
Quarry Bay

2562 7901

The Thai Café offers good Thai food in a down-to-earth, casual style. Like everywhere else in Quarry Bay, this place is extremely busy during the lunch hours so is best enjoyed in the evening time.

The menu provides a spice monitor to help you choose dishes depending on your taste. There is a range of dishes for $60 or less, including tom yum kung for $50; red, green and yellow curries for $60; phat Thai for $55; and deep fried spring rolls for $40. The meals are nicely presented and tasty.

The portions could be larger for the price but, overall, it's not a bad place to sample some tasty Thai food in a relaxed atmosphere.

Thai Orchids

G/F, 39 Tong Chong St.,
Taikoo Place,
Quarry Bay

2856 9848

Hours:
12pm-12am daily

Takeaway: Yes
Credit Cards: V, MC,AE

The Thai Orchids Café and Bar receives mixed reviews, ranging from 'I don't go anywhere else' to 'It's nothing special'. It's a fact that the prices inside the restaurant are relatively expensive but, don't despair, there's a takeaway section at the back of the restaurant offering cheaper fare.

Some reasonably priced dishes indoors include the fried seasonal vegetables with salted fish and garlic for $55 and the charcoal grilled chicken with Thai herbs for $60. Around the back though, most of the takeaway meals are priced at $44. This includes the very hot red curry chicken with rice, fried flat noodles with spicy minced beef, and the yellow curry ox-brisket with rice.

So, now that you are equipped with the facts, visit the inside restaurant or takeaway section and decide for yourself.

Vietnamese Food

Hours:
M to Sa: 10.30am-9.30pm
Su & PH: Closed

Takeaway: Yes
Credit Cards: None

G/F, 9 Hoi Kwong Street,
Quarry Bay

2811 2159

The Vietnamese Food House is packed out at lunchtimes and adequately fulfils the (office-worker) patrons' requirements - quick, standard size and quality, and good priced food. Come in the evening if you want to relax and enjoy the Vietnamese food, décor and bamboo chairs in a less busy environment.

The menu is extensive and the prices are relatively cheap. Cold noodle dishes cost up to $30; noodles in soup average $25; and the chef's special dishes (the main courses) are mostly $40. Further, fried chicken in leaves is $32; beef cube, French style, is $40; and a range of rolls is $28.

The food is what you'd expect for the prices, but that's okay if you're looking for a cheap meal with a wide choice of dishes.

Palm Court Cafe

Shop G110 of the
Repulse Bay Arcade,
109 Repulse Bay Rd,
Repulse Bay

2812-2903

Hours:
M to F: 11am-6pm
Sa to Su: 8:30am-6:30pm
PH: 10am-6:30pm
Takeaway: Yes
Credit Cards: AE,V,D,MC

Like the Repulse Bay Arcade complex that it is
housed in, the Palm Court Café appears
expensive and possibly off-limits to the hungry
but price-conscious general public. But that is not
actually the case and decent priced, good quality
food, served by efficient and polite staff, awaits
the diner in one of Hong Kong's most pleasant
surroundings.

The Palm Court Café is a delightful café with
seating either inside in the small shop or outside
in the courtyard at round tables under big
umbrellas.   Everything on the menu is around
$30 and this includes soup, salads and some
interesting sandwiches (both the latter come pre-
prepared). There are also afternoon tea sets,
plus you can get bread, pastries, cakes and good
coffee.

Come here to people-watch on a sunny day!

Chinese   **Tai Fat Hau**

Hours:
9am–3am daily

Sea View Building,
16 Beach Road,
Repulse Bay

Takeaway: Yes
Credit Cards: V,MC,AE

2812 2113

There are four terms to describe this restaurant - location, location, location and 'in need of a face lift'.

Tai Fat Hau, located right on the edge of the beach at Repulse Bay, yawns of a grander past. There are two menus - an expensive one and a cheaper, smaller one - so it's worth asking for the latter if it's not already on your table. The food is very local and is split into the usual main menu areas of rice and noodle dishes. Diced pork with sweetcorn is $55 and so too is the sliced beef rice noodle. Noodles in soup, for example the mixed pork or preserved vegetable, average $38. There's also a BBQ area open during busy holiday times.

The food may not be the tastiest or cheapest local fare around, but with outside terrace seating overlooking the beach, it's worth coming here just for a drink.

Happy Garden   Vietnamese / Thai

786 Shek O Village,
Shek O

Hours:
11am–11pm daily

2809 4165

Takeaway: Yes
Credit Cards: None

If you feel like Vietnamese food, then this is the
place to visit if you are in the area.

There's also a selection of tasty Thai meals listed
on the most professional looking menu in town.
Chicken, beef and pork dishes cost up to $55 and
vegetarian dishes average $45 each. Or for
something really cheap, don't miss the
Vietnamese cold noodles for $28.

When it comes to seafood, fried mussels with
curry or squid is $60, and a small spicy and sour
fish soup is also $60.

The restaurant has a view only over the car park,
but if you look hard enough you may just glimpse
the sea.

Hours: 303 Shek O Village,
11.30am–10pm daily   **Shek O**

Takeaway: Yes
Credit Cards: AE,V,MC   2809 4426

Shek O Chinese and Thailand Seafood Restaurant
is the most popular restaurant in Shek O, frequented by hikers, swimmers and more leisurely
weekend day-trippers. Like the other restaurants
in Shek O, the décor is nothing flash but there's
plenty of outdoor seating and large tables to cater
for groups.

The menu is also large with reasonable prices.
For example, steamed mussels with garlic, and
fried squid or shrimps with chili and basil, are
available for $55.

Other fish dishes are $70 or more but, don't
worry, this seafood restaurant doesn't offer only
seafood. Fried beef with black bean sauce is $50
and fried chicken with cashew is $55. Vegetarian
dishes, for example the fried mixed vegetable
with curry, average $45 each.

While the food is not absolutely fantastic here, it's
okay, and worth a visit if you're in town.

Welcome Garden   Asian

770 Shek O Village,   **Hours:**
Shek O   11:30am-10:30pm daily

2809 2836   **Takeaway:** Yes
                                    Credit Cards: None

Located opposite the Shek O Chinese and
Thailand Seafood Restaurant, this place has the
same look and feel as the others in Shek O, but
with its main food attraction being the varied
range of Asian dishes.

While Welcome Garden offers mostly Chinese
cuisine - for example, fried noodle with sliced
squid is $38 - there is also rijstafel and other non-
local items on the menu. These include sautéed
beef with chili sauce, and stir fried sliced chicken,
both for $58, throwing the cuisine type into the
'Asian' basket.

Probably the best difference about this restaurant
is that it offers free parking, which is a bonus,
especially on a Sunday when parking spaces are
hard to come by.

Cafe   **Balcony Cafe**

Hours: 203-204, 2/F,
9am–8pm daily   Stanley Plaza,
                                                      Stanley

Takeaway: Yes
Credit Cards: None   2813 5386

The Balcony café is actually an extension of
Stanley's Park n' Shop and you can enter either
through the supermarket or from the outside via a
lift from the Plaza.

The prices are cheap (everything is under $40)
and the food is standard café fare. You can
choose sandwiches for $34 that come served with
meat, salad and a choice of bread; pasta for $32;
and meat pies for $21. There are also breakfast,
lunch and tea sets that are reasonably priced, and
you can sit either inside or outside - both with a
view over the square.

And, keeping in line with enterprising cafés the
world over, there are even a couple of computers
providing twenty minutes of free Internet access
with any purchase over $30.

Chilli n' Spice

Shop No. 101,
Murray House,
Stanley Plaza,
Stanley

2899 0147

Hours:
M to Sa: 12am–11.30pm
Su: 11am–11pm

Takeaway: Yes
Credit Cards: V,MC,AE

Located on the second floor of the impressive colonial edifice of Murray House, Chilli n' Spice offers Asian style food and balcony seating with a view over Stanley Main Street and the sea.

The food quality and prices are impressive for such a location. The Indonesian curry brisket or chicken and the sweet and sour pork rib are both $50. For vegetarians, the sautéed mixed vegetables Thai style is $45 and, for those wanting seafood, the Indonesian seafood fried rice is $58.

Its sister restaurant in Discovery Bay also offers a fine sea view but not the shaded and breezy balcony seating that is a key selling point for this location.

See the Branches section for other restaurants in the group.

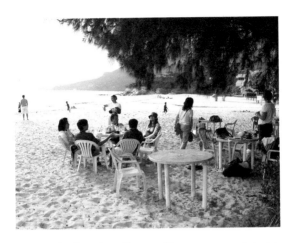

▲ Eat on the beach - Cheung Sha (PHOTO: Nicole Lade)
▼ Grab a bite near the beach - Shek O (PHOTO: Iris Cheung)

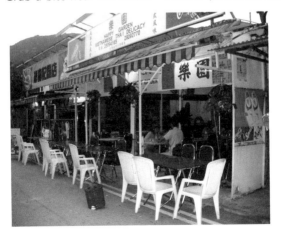

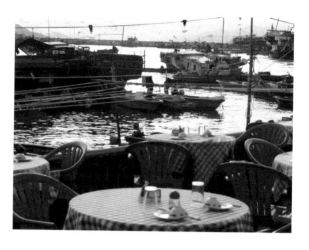

▲ Cheung Chau harbour (PHOTO: Kylie Uebergang)
▼ Fish balls by the scoopful (PHOTO: Kylie Uebergang)

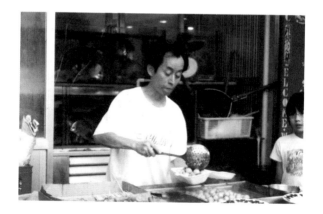

Pub

Lord Stanley's

Hours:
M to F: 10am-1am
Sa & Su: 9am-1am

Takeaway: Yes
Credit Cards: V,AE

G/F, 92A Stanley Main
Street,
Stanley

2813 0993

The décor at the Lord Stanley is a cross between a pub found in beachside England and a roadside diner in the United States, but the food is good pub grub.

Most of the main dishes are $65 or more but there are a range of soups, salads, sandwiches and snacks that are cheaper at $60 or less. The BLT is huge and tasty at $50, while the Shanghai prawn dumplings soup is an okay attempt at local fare for $52. A Caesar salad is available at $58, and the interesting onion soup with stilton cheese is $44 for a cup and $52 for a bowl.

The Lord Stanley is not a bad place to while away a few pub hours watching the football inside or the world go by from the tables outside.

New Star

Upper G/F, 40-42
Stanley Main Street,
Stanley

2813 9982

Stanley

Hours:
8am-8pm daily

Takeaway: Yes
Credit Cards: None

There are some good local restaurants located in Stanley Market and this is one of them.

Popular with the locals, the New Star offers a range of rice, curry pot and noodle dishes as well as sandwiches and snacks, all for $45 or less. For example, stewed beef and vegetable with rice is $32; chicken and seasonal vegetable fried noodle is $35; garoupa curry with rice is $40; and shrimp dumpling noodle soup is $18. The most expensive dishes are the roasted spare ribs and the satay sticks (chicken or beef) for $45.

Most seating is inside but there is also some seating in the narrow alleyway outside.

Thai / Chinese **Stanley Restaurant**

Hours:
7am–10.30pm daily

Upper G/F,
52-56 Stanley Main St.,
Stanley

Takeaway: Yes
Credit Cards: None

2813 7998

Offering Thai as well as Chinese fare, this busy restaurant is especially popular with the locals. While some dishes are expensive, particularly the Thai seafood, prices are generally reasonable at the Stanley Restaurant.

All the curry colours are available with pork, beef or chicken for $45; rice dishes average $30, for example, rice with fried garoupa; and fried noodles range from $30 to $45. 'Casserole food' or hotpots are also available, for example, seafood with assorted vegetables in casserole is $42.

The food and prices at this place are a little more upmarket than other local restaurants in the market, but the choice of dishes and outside seating are what make it appealing.

Thai Thai

5/F, 90B Stanley Main
St.,
Stanley

2813 7818

Hours:
M to Sa: 11.45am-3pm
& 6pm-11pm
Sa & Su: 11.45pm-11pm
Takeaway: Yes
Credit Cards: V,MC,AE,D

Located five floors up, Thai Thai offers good views
over the sea in a modern, fine-dining-ambience
restaurant. White linen tablecloths and napkins
are found on the tables giving the impression that
prices will be high. But not all of them are and
you can enjoy the fine food, service and
atmosphere here without breaking the bank.

From the Chef's Specialities menu, charcoal
grilled cuttlefish served with spicy and sour sauce
is $52, and the BBQ slice of pork neck served in
spicy sauce is also $52. Vegetarian dishes also
average around $52, for example, the fried mixed
vegetable with garlic and oyster sauce, or the
green curry with mixed vegetables. Noodle
dishes are around $48 and salads are priced up to
$58.

If you feel like authentic Thai, in a smart
restaurant, Thai Thai is the place to go. (Also at
G/F, 3 Lan Fong Road, Causeway Bay, 2895
0699).

Pub   **The Smuggler's Inn**

Hours: G/F, 90A Stanley Main St.,
10am-12am daily   **Stanley**

Takeaway: Yes
Credit Cards: V,MC   2813 8852

Full of British tourists during the weekdays and expat locals on the weekend, The Smuggler's Inn is a traditional look-and-feel English pub. It offers food but the kitchen closes at 7pm and there's no table service. Seating is on small stools and at small tables inside or on high bench seating outside.

The food is exactly what you'd expect from an English pub. You can choose from a range of pies, served with beans, mushy peas or salad, for $45, or the steak sandwich served with sautéed mushrooms and onions for $40. If they don't tempt you, then there's the hot dog served with salad and hot dog relish for $35, or salads or submarines served with meat or fish and salad 'fillings' for a similar price.

While the food is very 'pubby', the Smuggler's Inn is really more of a drinker's pub. Either way it's a great place to enjoy a piece of England.

The Wok   Asian

G/F, 14–14A Stanley
Main Street,
Stanley

Hours:
10am–10pm daily

Takeaway: Yes
2813 9787   **Credit Cards:** V,MC

The cuisine type at The Wok is 'Asian' but it would
be more appropriately described as 'Western style
Asian'. Located smack-bang in the middle of the
market, with raised outside seating, you can't
beat the location for a bite while shopping.

The menu covers the gamut of Asian dishes from
gado gado ($60) and tom yum seafood soup
($55) to chicken tikka ($60), but with a few
decidedly non-Asian dishes, for example,
vegetarian spaghetti ($60) and fish and chips
($70).

There's no MSG used in the cooking but the food
has a distinctly Western taste. Check it out for
the choice of Western and Asian dishes.

American   **EAT (on ice)**

Hours:
M to F: 11:30am-10pm
Sa to Su: 9am-10pm

Shop 136, 1/F, Cityplaza,
18 Taikoo Shing Road,
Taikoo Shing

Takeaway: Yes
Credit Cards: V,MC,AE

2567 8608

EAT (on ice) is literally that. Unique in Hong Kong, the American-diner style restaurant is situated alongside an ice-skating rink in Taikoo Shing's Cityplaza shopping centre. Diners can enjoy a view of the skaters, and skaters can skate in and out to get food and drinks without having to take their skates off.

Most of the food is diner-style - similar to the other EAT in Pacific Place - and you can order snacks and appetisers, like French fries for $26, or sandwiches, hotdogs and burgers, such as the BBQ bacon cheese burger for $58. There are also salads, soups, pasta, Asian delights, desserts, drinks and a kid's menu to choose from.

The meal portions are generous, and the prices are not bad.

Bring the kids here for a somewhat different day out.

The Castle Restaurant International

G/F, Shop 402–403,
Yen Kung Mansions,
1 Tai Mou Avenue,
Taikoo Shing

2568 9808

Hours:
11am–11.30pm daily

Takeaway: Yes
Credit Cards: V,MC,AE

Located amongst the pillars of humanity that form
Taikoo Shing - just near Cityplaza - the Castle
Restaurant offers a range of Western style dishes
in a supposedly castle-like setting. The restaurant
is extremely busy during lunchtimes, catering
particularly to white-collar workers and, overall,
the food is okay.

The prices are reasonable for the area and for the
type and quality of food on offer. Pasta or rice
with pork, chicken, beef or lamb is $60; salads,
seafood or chicken dishes are $52; and lunch
sets, including the curry lamb or shrimp set (with
soup and tea or coffee) is $56. Steak on a hot
plate is $80 or more.

The Castle Restaurant provides a decent and
comfortable place for dining, particularly for
dinner when it is less crowded.

EAT Noodles

Hours:
M to Th: 11:30am-9:30pm
F & Sa: 11:30am-10pm
Su: 11:30am-9pm
Takeaway: Yes
Credit Cards: None

2/F Peak Tower,
128 Peak Road,
The Peak

2849 5777

The Peak

The EAT Noodles restaurant at this popular tourist location boasts an outdoor terrace seating area with sensational views over Hong Kong, and reasonable food prices.

All noodle dishes, whether in soup or broth or wok-tossed and stir-fried, are $38. For example, the Chinese roast duck and char siu with Hokkien noodles comes fast and tasty and is enjoyed even more while sitting outside taking in the view.

The location and prices are some of the best at the Peak, and the food's not too bad either.

Grappa's Peak Pizzeria   Italian

4/F, The Peak Tower,   **Hours:**
128 Peak Road,   10am-10pm daily
The Peak

                                     Takeaway: Yes
2849 4222   **Credit Cards:** V,MC,D

The most expensive items on the menu at
Grappa's Peak Pizzeria are the company's
memorabilia. The food here is relatively cheap
compared to other eateries at the Peak; for
example, you can choose from fettucine,
spaghetti or penne pasta with a range of sauce
toppings from $42 to $55.

A slice of daily pizza will set you back $25 or $35
for the standard or deluxe variety respectively,
and individual size pizzas range from $45 to $60.
Large pizzas are more expensive ($75 to $95) but
could easily be shared. You can also get snacks,
hamburgers and sandwiches here, all for under
$45. But the best thing about this restaurant, if
the prices have not enticed you enough, is that
there is seating available outside.

While the restaurant does not offer a view over
Hong Kong, it is a pleasant dining experience
nonetheless.

International   **Movenpick Marche**

Hours:
M to F: 11am-11pm
Sa & Su: 9am-11pm

Takeaway: No
Credit Cards: None

Level 6 & 7,
The Peak Tower,
128 Peak Road,
The Peak

2849 2000

The Movenpick Marche Restaurant bills itself as 'Hong Kong's highest restaurant' and it offers undeniably superb views over Hong Kong.

The restaurant is market style, as its French name suggests, and you can order meals from various 'market vendors' which are then cooked fresh in front of you.

There are plenty of market stalls to choose from, offering a range of food including noodles, pasta, seafood and meats (from the grill), sushi and fresh juices. Noodles are possibly the cheapest item on offer at around $30; pizzas are $48 or more; and pasta is on average $60 per meal. The meat and seafood dishes are generally priced a little higher again.

For The Peak, the food is not too badly priced, it's a novel dining experience, and you can't beat the view.

Cafe Loyal   Chinese

107 Wanchai Road,   **Hours:**
Wanchai   11:30am-11:30pm

                                      Takeaway: Yes
2574 8161   **Credit Cards:** None

Café Loyal sits a couple of rungs above the
standard dai pai dong. This becomes obvious
when you read the menu and see that wine is
available and that the prices are generally higher
than other restaurants in the neighbourhood.

Don't get too excited by the wine though -
although it's relatively cheap at $12 by the glass
or $60 per bottle, the quality is not the best. All
the meals, including the pork chop 'zizzling' plate
dish, come with a drink and are priced in the
$60+ range. There's a $48 meal deal that's not
bad value which includes Russian borsch or cream
soup, fried rice with smoked salmon and diced
chicken and pineapple, and tea or coffee. Even
better are the tea-time meals for $25. The
addition of the drink or soup in the prices is a
bonus but, overall, the restaurant is a little higher
priced than it can really justify.

Go for the tea-time set when you can almost have
the restaurant to yourself.

Chinese / Veg.

Healthy Mess

Hours:
M to Sa: 10:30am-11pm
Su: Closed

51-53 Hennessy Road,
Wanchai

Takeaway: Yes
Credit Cards: V,MC

2527 3918

The Healthy Mess Vegetarian Kitchen is a great vegetarian find in Wanchai. The food and service consistently receive rave reviews - not only is the food delicious, but also the staff are friendly and attentive.

Being a sister of the Nice Fragrance Vegetarian Kitchen (also reviewed), the menu is the same but with seasonal additions. Noodles generally range from $45 to $50 and main dishes start at $48. Thick vegetable soup, and the fried rice with cashew nuts, mixed vegetables and currants both ooze healthiness at $30 and $60 respectively. Other vegetarian delights are available for takeaway from the window counter at the front of the restaurant.

If you prefer vegetarian food or are in need of a dose of health, look no further than this great restaurant.

Queens Road East,
Wanchai

Hours:
10am-10pm daily

Takeaway: Yes
Credit Cards: None

Hong Kong is blessed with numerous outlets selling fresh fruit and vegetable juice - a great healthy alternative to the artificial supermarket variety.

Generally, juices in Hong Kong range from $10 to $15 for a standard size, depending on the ingredients, but on Queen's Road East, Wanchai, a price war has pushed prices even lower. All juices go for under $10 - you'll find apple or orange juices priced for just $5 and mango juice for a low $8.

It's worth taking a detour to any of these shops along Queens Road East, starting from near the Wanchai wet market, to experience cheap fruit juice at its best.

Indian

Jo Jo Mess Club

Hours:
12pm-3pm
& 6pm-11pm daily

1/F, 86 Johnston Road,
Wanchai

Takeaway: Yes
Credit Cards: V,MC,D,AE

2527 3776

Jo Jo Mess Club has all the trimmings of Indian restaurants in Hong Kong. The entrance is an insalubrious stairwell, the food is served by Indian staff, there's Indian music playing, and the décor is typically unimpressive. But there are a couple of different characteristics here - most of the patrons are non-Indian and the food is not so authentic-tasting.

All the usual Indian dishes are available though and the prices are reasonable at around the $50 mark for most meals. The navrattan korma is $42 and comes with plentiful spices - perhaps to mask the seemingly 'out-of-the-can' vegetables included in the dish.

However, there are some redeeming qualities which make a visit to the restaurant worthwhile if you are in the area. That is, the view is good (overlooking the busy Southorn sportsground), the staff are friendly and the beer is cheaper than the soft drinks. See the Branches section for other locations.

King of the Beef

206 Johnston Road,
Wanchai

Hours:
7am-1am daily

2573 1083

Takeaway: Yes
Credit Cards: None

King of the Beef does not offer only steaks or
meat dishes as the name might suggest. In fact,
it offers noodle and rice dishes like many other
small restaurants around. The main difference is
the industrial-style décor - that is, the walls are
concrete and if you look up you can see the
plumbing and all.

The food is nothing special but it's okay for the
price. Some of the fare and prices on offer
include: baked rice dishes, for example the baked
sliced steak with satay sauce and rice, ranging
from $33 to $38; boiled rice sets, for example,
pork with XO sauce, for $31 (including a drink);
and the Japanese style eel rice bowl for $29.

But the clincher is that the 'special' is baked
seafood with rice (for $38), prompting one to ask:
shouldn't this place be called 'King of the Reef'
instead?

Hours:
8am-8pm daily

Urban Services Complex,
225 Hennessy Road,
Wanchai

Takeaway: Yes
Credit Cards: None

There's one of these 'dai pai dongs' in every district (usually located above the wet market) and if you want a cheap, fresh meal - local style - then these are the places to come to. The Lockhart Road Market Food Court is no exception.

Located above the market, it's loud and crowded and you'll most likely have to wait for, and then share, a table at lunchtime. It has about 10 different outlets that all merge into one, each differentiated by the colour of their chopsticks and the slightly different fare. One of the shops, translated loosely as 'Char Kee', offers delicious food. The soup with fish and bak choy has a very tasty lemongrass flavour, and comes with a big bowl of rice and soy sauce for only $22. For $19, they offer a tasty fish and dark egg congee, also with soy sauce on the side.

No one speaks English, but it's a great place to sample some of the cheapest and freshest food around.

New Derby

Pub

Wanchai

Shop G-1, G/F,
Valley Centre,
80-82 Morrison Hill Road,
Wanchai

2893 9123

Hours:
12pm-2am daily

Takeaway: Yes
Credit Cards: V,MC

Located within stumbling distance from the Happy Valley racetrack, the New Derby offers a big screen for sport lovers, a turntable for music lovers and some pub grub for food lovers (or for those who are just hungry).

The food is typical pub fare at fairly reasonable prices. From the main menu on the bar you can choose from spring rolls for $25; beer battered fish and chips for $42; or tenderloin with black pepper and onion for $38. There is also a blackboard offering daily specials, including baked pork chop with rice ($58), that come with soup and a drink.

The pub has a good atmosphere - it's small with dark wood panelling and floorboards, and comfortable bench seats - and you won't go hungry after a day or night at the races.

Chinese / Veg.

Nice Fragrance

Hours:
M to F: 10.30am-11pm
Sa & Su: 8am-9pm

Takeaway: Yes
Credit Cards: AE,V,MC,D

105-107 Thomson Road,
Wanchai

2838 3067

The Nice Fragrance Vegetarian Kitchen presents Buddhist calm among dining madness. With a shrine in the corner, pictures of Buddha lining the walls and Buddhist memorabilia available for sale, this restaurant is a bigger and busier branch of the Healthy Mess Vegetarian Kitchen (also reviewed).

There are 116 items on the menu and, with each of them, you can actually taste the freshness of the vegetables. Not following the Hong Kong mantra of 'all vegetables = choi sum', you'll be pleasantly surprised to see fresh snowpeas, carrots, mushrooms, tofu and the like on the menu.

The fried rice is possibly the best to be found in Hong Kong - extremely tasty and not oily. Prices generally start at $40 and go up from there.

O Tree Caffe and Bar

Cafe

Shop G4,
Sun Hung Kai Centre,
Wanchai

2877 7009

Hours:
M to Sa: 7am-7pm
Su: Closed

Takeaway: Yes
Credit Cards: V,MC

The O Tree Caffe & Bar looks a little bit like a bar but its menu is 100% café fare. Either way, it's quite comfortable (albeit dimly-lit), it's decorated in a modern cream, orange and brown colour-scheme and offers cushioned seating.

All the usual café (not bar) items are available including non-alcoholic drinks, salads, soup, pasta, rice and sandwiches. Most main meal dishes are around the $48 mark or more, including the smoked salmon with herbs cream sauce pasta for $58, and the roast beef sandwich, with black pepper, mustard and pickles, for $48.

Don't be confused by the name - the O Tree Caffe & Bar is not a bad place to sit and relax, and get an okay café style meal, but a lively bar it is not.

Thai   **Pad Thai**

Hours: 2/F, One Capital Place,
M to F: 12pm-3pm   18 Luard Road,
& 6pm-12am   **Wanchai**
Sa & Su: 12pm-12am
Takeaway: Yes
Credit Cards: MC,V,AE,D   2126 7900

Pad Thai offers delicious and authentic Thai food
in a modern and stylish restaurant. It's located
above Delaney's Irish Bar and caters well for
large and small groups alike.

One would expect the expensive-looking décor
found here to equate to higher prices but this is
not particularly the case. Thai fish cakes are not
too oily at $52; the pad Thai comes wrapped in
omelette for $54; and the chicken curry is deli-
cious at $58. Just to keep those taste buds
juicing, the grilled marinated pork pieces are
tender at $56 and, if you feel like a splurge, the
raw baby prawns marinated in lime, nam pla and
chili are an absolute must at $70.

The best thing to do is come here with a group so
that you can taste many dishes at the same time,
or just keep coming back to try more.

Pho Saigon — Vietnamese

G/F, 319 Hennessy Road,
Wanchai

Hours:
11am-12:30am daily

2833 6833

Takeaway: Yes
Credit Cards: None

With another branch in Mongkok (at G/F, 224A Fa Yuen Street, Mongkok, 2142 7747), Pho Saigon offers simple and tasty Vietnamese fare in a clean, unpretentious environment.

With Vietnamese music softly playing, the friendly staff will happily provide you upon request with the one English menu. Prices are cheap with every dish under $39. For example, pho with lean beef is $29; all cold vermicelli 'bun' dishes are $34; spring rolls are $29; and rice dishes, including chicken curry with steamed rice, are $34. The afternoon tea set offers similar dishes at even cheaper prices.

For a taste of Vietnam in a down-to-earth setting, venture no further than Pho Saigon.

Indian

Shaffi's Malik

Hours:
12pm-3pm
& 6pm-11pm daily

Takeaway: Yes
Credit Cards: V,MC,D,AE

G/F, Connaught
Commercial Building,
185 Wanchai Road,
Wanchai

2572 7474

Run by a Pakistani, Shaffi's Malik Restaurant is 'probably the oldest Indian restaurant in Hong Kong' - allegedly. The restaurant has interesting décor with wood panelling, booth seats down one side and dimmed lighting. The food, however, is not dim.

The navrattan korma is sweet in taste and price at $52, and the beef vindaloo is hot in taste and price at $58. Tandoori specialities are $58, the chicken korma is $50 and the mutton bhunna goes for $50.

Kingfisher beer is available and a video plays Bollywood films to add to the atmosphere. Definitely a restaurant worth trying.

Shanghai Food　　　　　Chinese

G/F, 218 Wanchai Road,
Wanchai

Hours:
11am-11:30pm daily

2573 8973

Takeaway: Yes
Credit Cards: V,MC

This restaurant serves great food and is certainly worth a visit. If you can't speak Cantonese, it may be worth taking a local speaker along with you, because there's no English menu. But that adds to the adventure and you won't be disappointed.

The following dishes come recommended: dam dam noodles - thin noodles in a slightly spicy peanut sauce - for $24; ten pork dumplings with soy and chili dipping sauces for $37; and fried pork with thick Shanghai noodles in soy sauce for $30. It's the kind of place where your tea glass is constantly refilled and you can slop away to your heart's content.

The décor is interesting: floral wallpaper, a huge antique mirror and velvet seats. This, along with the delicious food, good prices and the opera singing waitress, all add up to a great experience.

International **Tiffany Restaurant**

Hours:
8am–11.30pm daily

188 Hennessy Road,
Wanchai

Takeaway: Yes
Credit Cards: V,MC,AE

2381 1516

The Tiffany Restaurant is quite unique for Wanchai. On arrival, it's reminiscent of stepping into your grandma's house - with floral carpet, floral padded seats and booths, tea served in a pot, and a general feeling of space and geniality not normally found in this part of town.

There's an unexpectedly diverse menu which includes shashlik of kangaroo and roast ostrich steak, and proper waiter service too. Prices vary and include spaghetti bolognaise for $55, which is served with baked cheese, diced carrot and peas on top; beef stroganoff also for $55; and the curry vegetable and egg for $50. Soups and salads are some of the cheaper items and the tea set (from 2.45pm to 6pm) also includes a large serving of special fried noodles for $38.

While the food is okay, it's really the quiet and relaxed atmosphere you come here for. They also have a branch in Mongkok - see the Branches section for details.

Tomozuna   Japanese

Unit E, G/F,
283 Hennessy Road,
Wanchai

2583 9770

Hours:
11am-3pm
& 6pm-11.45am daily

Takeaway: Yes
Credit Cards: V,MC

The Tomozuna Restaurant is located on the unofficial 'Japanese row' - a strip along Hennessy Road in Wanchai where many Japanese restaurants have congregated.

You can sit at the counter watching the chefs do their stuff or at small tables and, either way, you'll be impressed by the joviality and friendliness of the staff. There are a range of dishes available, including ramens, with a choice of soup base, for $29 to $48 (the vegetable ramen is tasty and healthy at $35); rice dishes, for example, salmon in soup with rice for $40; and freshly prepared sushi and sashimi which starts at around $20 for two pieces of red tuna roll. Fried or cold noodles, fried rice and grilled dishes are also available.

If Japanese is your food preference, then you won't be disappointed by a visit to Tomozuna.

Cafe   **Zambra**

Hours:
7am-7pm daily

13 O'Brien Road
& 239 Jaffe Road,
Wanchai

Takeaway: No
Credit Cards: Yes

2802 2226/2598 1322

There are two Zambras quite close to each other in Wanchai. One is a little hole-in-the-wall coffee shop located underneath the walking overpass to the Government offices, and the other is a relatively new café situated on Jaffe Road. Both are worth knowing about, especially for their 'foreigner-friendly' food and drink offerings which are a bit unique in this very Chinese part of town.

The hole-in-the-wall Zambra specialises in coffees, which are around $19 each, but it also offers nicely-made sandwiches for $26, salads-to-go for $35 and a selection of muffins. There are a couple of bench seats and newspapers to read but this is really a takeaway shop.

The other Zambra, the café down the road, is quite large with modern décor and comfortable seating. There's a large selection of salads, all around $18 to $25 per serving, as well as cakes, desserts, bakery items and, of course, the signature coffee that you can enjoy sitting in.

Kowloon

Kowloon is a bargain hunter's paradise and this is equally true for the food on offer. Cheap eats can be found everywhere – in particular in Tsim Sha Tsui, Jordan, Kowloon City and Hung Hom - and the restaurants' cuisines serve diners of all walks of life who call this area home or who work and play here.

Chungking Mansions, Katiga Street and Temple Street are all renowned budget eating areas in Kowloon. The infamous Chungking Mansions, in Tsim Sha Tsui, is home to a wide array of great value restaurants serving Indian and Pakistani cuisine. Katiga Street is a hidden haven of Japanese fare tucked away in the alleyways on and off Sung Kit Street in Hung Hom, and Temple Street, in Jordan, is not only home to the well known night market but also to a host of cheap, local style restaurants. Little known Hau Fook Street, in Tsim Sha Tsui, is also a budget dining enclave particularly patronised by the locals.

Katiga Street

Japanese

G/F, Sung Oi Building,
37 Sung Kit Street,
Hung Hom

Hours:
11.30am-11.00pm daily

2764 6436

Takeaway: Yes
Credit Cards: V,MC,AE,D

Tucked away in the alleyways on and off Sung Kit Street in Hung Hom is a hidden haven of Japanese fare known as Katiga Street. While the official restaurant name is Katiga Japanese Food Shop, there are actually a few shops (or restaurants) that share the same kitchen and facilities and go by the same name. The décor is Japanese kitsch and, interestingly, the staff who prepare food wear mouth masks.

It's definitely a feast for the eyes and not a bad feast for the stomach either. Salads, such as the crab roe Japanese salad, are around $35, vegetable tempura is $38 and Japanese dishes, such as smoked duck and grilled sea eel liver, are $45. Sharing an enormous bowl of noodles ($128) with friends is one of Katiga's key attractions, and there are a number of set meals available for less than $60.

Katiga Street makes for a good night out, especially with a group of friends.

Hours: Temple Street,
12pm-12am daily   **Jordan**

Takeaway: Yes
Credit Cards: None

Temple Street is renowned as a bargain shopper's
paradise; the same goes for food. Not only does
Temple Street itself offer cheap dining but the
area immediately surrounding it also does.

The food is generally 100% local style with dining
on plastic seats, and sometimes not under cover,
the norm. Two restaurants along Temple Street fit
the bill perfectly: Tak Kee Seafood Restaurant and
Wing Fat Seafood Restaurant. Both offer similar
fare and it's easy to eat well – ordering such
dishes as steamed fish, and Chinese vegetables
with beef - for around $40. Restaurants along
Temple Street generally offer cheaper beer too.

Look for the night market and you know you've
found Temple Street; then look for painted menus
and you know you've found some of the cheapest
restaurants around.

Traditional Noodle

Chinese

53 Pilkem Street,
Jordan

Hours:
11am–11pm daily

2730 8200

Takeaway: Yes
Credit Cards: None

Located near the madness of Temple Street, but far enough away to feel more local and calm, the Traditional Chinese Noodle shop is a small eatery which offers build-your-own noodle dishes as its speciality.

The flavoursome 'base' dish (broth and noodles of varying degrees of spiciness) costs $17, and then it's a matter of adding as few or as many 'extras' as you like, for $3 each. The 'extras' include all the usuals such as wontons, fish balls, spicy vegetables and shredded chicken. There are also ready-made noodle dishes that you can choose from, ranging up to $30.

Drop by the Traditional Chinese Noodle shop if you are feeling a bit picky about what goes in your noodle dish, and you won't be disappointed.

Thai   **Friendship Thai**

Hours: G/F, 38 Kai Tak Road,
11am-11pm daily   **Kowloon City**

Takeaway: Yes
Credit Cards: V,MC   2382 8671

Located in once-bustling Kowloon City, Friendship
Thai is in the middle of a light industrial area that
may not be normally associated with good food.
But Thai restaurants abound here, where the
international airport used to be, and the
Friendship Thai restaurant is hailed as one of the
area's best.

With a tri-lingual menu, the clientele is a mixed
bunch of regulars - including Thai workers, locals
and 'gweilos' - which is the first proof of its
authenticity. The second is that the staff are all
Thai. But the resounding proof is the food. The
Thai style vegetarian hotpot, for $49, is tasty and
filling. In general the prices are reasonable:
pork, beef and chicken dishes are priced in the
$50s, and vegetable dishes in the $40s.

The Friendship Thai is definitely worth seeking out
if you happen to find yourself hungry in Kowloon
City.

Jane Kee

Thai

Shop #20,
57–67C Kai Tin Road,
Lam Tin

2717 4839

Hours:
9am-11pm daily

Takeaway: Yes
Credit Cards: None

Being a primarily Chinese residential area in Kowloon, Lam Tin is not the kind of place you'd expect to find a Thai restaurant. Accordingly, the owners haven't prepared for English-speaking clientele and you'll find only a Chinese menu in a very local style restaurant. But, if you are in the area, Jane Kee is worth a look because the prices are cheap and the food is tasty and served in generous portions.

The Thai style fried rice is $30, fried rice with seafood is $30, fried pork in pepper and garlic sauce is $40, and tom yam soup is $35 for a small and $60 for a large. The spices are very Thai but not too hot so the food can be enjoyed by all palates.

Jane Kee is a good place to visit with a group of people so that you can try a range of dishes - but just make sure that one of your party can speak Cantonese.

Indian   **Afghan Canteen**

Hours: Wing Lok Building, 3/F,
M to Sa: 12.30pm-2.30pm   14A Peking Road,
& 6pm-11pm   **Tsim Sha Tsui**
Su: 6pm-11pm
Takeaway: Yes
Credit Cards: None   2367 7489

If you like hot, spicy Indian food, then the Afghan Canteen will not disappoint you. Even though the menu asks you to state your taste preference to the waiter, don't be surprised if you ask for 'mild' and it tastes more like 'medium'.

Spiciness aside, the food here is fantastic, the service is good and it's one of those places that, once you've found it (note that the entrance is on Lock Road), you'll keep loyally returning. And the prices are reasonable too. Tandoori specialities start at $54, chicken dishes (including the very hot chicken vindaloo) are around the $56 mark, and vegetable curries are $44.

Make sure you leave enough room to try the malai kulfi (homemade Indian ice cream) for $18 - it's a delicious dish to top off your meal with (and might help to cool down your mouth).

Branto

Indian

1/F, 9 Lock Road,
Tsim Sha Tsui

Hours:
6pm-12am daily

Takeaway: Yes
Credit Cards: V,MC

2366 8171

Don't be put off by the inconspicuous entrance; Branto is definitely worth a visit, particularly if you are a fan of authentic Indian vegetarian food.

The fact that the majority of its customers are Indian is a sure sign that the restaurant has got the food, service and price right. And that they have - the food, in particular, constantly receives rave reviews. As an example of the menu offerings: the vegetable kadai is full of health at $57, the masala dosa is tasty at $29, and the special Indian thali for $55 is a great meal in itself.

The restaurant décor is typical Indian, and Bollywood song clips are played for your listening enjoyment, which only add positively to the overall must-try dining experience.

Vietnamese

Coconut Forest

Hours:
11:00am-12:30am daily

2 Hau Fook Street,
Tsim Sha Tsui

Takeaway: Yes
Credit Cards: V,MC

2312 0086

The pedestrianised Hau Fook Street is renowned as a bargain eating area, catering more to purveyors and diners of Chinese food. The Coconut Forest Vietnamese Restaurant is a welcome addition to the street, offering an undeniable taste of Vietnam.

Most dishes, including rice and noodles, are $38 but you will find other, more exotic delights on the menu, such as fried frog and peppermint for $60. Colourful fruit jelly desserts and coconuts, as the restaurant's name suggests, are also available.

Both are on display in the front glass window, standing out like a navigational beacon; look for them to help you find your way.

Edo Restaurant   Japanese

Shop 228, 2/F,
New World Centre,
24 Salisbury Road,
Tsim Sha Tsui

2367 7882

Hours:
10am-8:30pm daily

Takeaway: Yes
Credit Cards: None

Located at the back of the supermarket in the New World Centre, this Japanese restaurant is worth a visit if you are in the area shopping or staying nearby. It's quite unpretentious, occupies a large space (so you'll always get a seat), has friendly staff and the food isn't bad either.

The assorted vegetable ramen actually comes with a range of vegetables and is decently priced at $28. Other ramens range up to $38 and rice dishes are generally under $40. And then there's the a-la-carte menu where you can choose from a range of Japanese dishes, for example, the not-too-battered prawn with vegetables tempura, for less than $38.

The restaurant doesn't offer too much in the way of table service (you normally pay at the front counter before you eat), but with unlimited tea continuously topped up as you eat, this place won't break the bank.

Chinese   **Every Time Cafe**

Hours: G/F & 1/F,
7:30am-3am daily   22-24 Prat Avenue,
                                             Tsim Sha Tsui

Takeaway: Yes
Credit Cards: None   2721 3738

The Every Time Café is a modern, alternative
style café that seems to attract the groovy
Chinese set to its doors. Perhaps it's the
Burberry-covered booth seats or the guarantee of
MTV playing well into the night that's so appealing,
because the food and service receive mixed
reviews.

The prices are good though. Rice with various
Chinese barbecued meat dishes are
recommended and range from $28 to $32; noodle
dishes start at $18 and go up to $48; and other
main dishes are around $55. There are also
sandwiches, omelettes and toast, starting at $8, to
choose from.

So if you want to be part of the scene, this is a
good place to start (oh, and some style advice:
maybe leave your Burberry handbag at home so
that it doesn't clash with the seats).

Gig Restaurant International

8 Hart Avenue,
Tsim Sha Tsui

Hours:
12pm-12am daily

2316 9988

Takeaway: Yes
Credit Cards: V,MC,AE

Billed as a music café, the Gig Restaurant offers something a bit different to the standard T.S.T. dining experience. As well as offering a range of mainly Western style meals and snacks, served in a smart, classy-looking restaurant, there are also live bands playing almost every night.

The music is the number one draw card here with the invariably Chinese bands kicking off between 7.30pm and 10pm. The food and service, however, get mixed reviews - possibly depending on the music quality of that night! On average snacks are available for $40 and main meals, for example, pasta, are available for $58.

Check the band and time schedule out the front of the restaurant - you never know, you might witness the makings of the next Andy Lau.

Guangdong Barbecue

Hours:
7am-1am daily

G/F, Hankow Building,
43 Hankow Road,
Tsim Sha Tsui

Takeaway: Yes
Credit Cards: None

2735 5151

This place is about as local as you can get - not only in the food that is offered but also in the restaurant's name. It's popular with the locals which, of course, is always a good sign of cheap prices and good food.

The Cantonese BBQ dishes are the main items to come for. The honeyed roast pork is succulent at $28 (with rice and lettuce for $33); and larger rice dishes, including roast goose, start at $38. There are also noodle and main course dishes to choose from, including: fried noodle with beef and vegetables for $40; noodles in soup for an average $38 to $45; and sweet and sour garoupa, one of the most expensive items on the menu at $55.

Whether you're a tourist or a local, it's worth coming to the Guangdong Barbecue Restaurant to sample some typical Guangdong cuisine at decent prices.

Happy Garden

76 Canton Road,
Tsim Sha Tsui

Hours:
7am-12.30am daily

2377 2604

Takeaway: Yes
Credit Cards: None

The Happy Garden Noodle and Congee Kitchen is well known for offering cheap, local style food in a friendly and cosy atmosphere. Decorated in mock old-worldy Chinese décor, there are 200 menu items to choose from.

Keeping true to its name, noodles and congee are the specialities, and as an example of the food and prices on offer, the shrimp wonton noodles dish is $22, and various types of congee average around $30 a bowl. Vermicelli Singapore style is $33 and noodles with wonton and beef brisket in soup is $28. There are also some non-noodles and congee dishes to choose from, including the stir-fried sliced fillet of beef in oyster sauce for $55.

The staff make you feel very welcome and, with the cheap prices, it's an easy place to return to.

Indonesian   **Indonesia Restaurant**

Hours:
12pm-11:30pm daily

66 Granville Road,
Tsim Sha Tsui

Takeaway: Yes
Credit Cards: V,MC,D,AE

2367 3287

This is one of the best Indonesian restaurants in Hong Kong and consistently receives good reviews for both the food and service. Loyal customers have been patronizing the restaurant since its inception in 1971 and, even though it's large, it's recommended that you make a booking, especially if you are dining in the evening.

The food is as authentic as it gets, including karis (curries) priced up to $60 and nasi (rice) dishes ranging from $48 to $55. Wash it down with juice from a real coconut and take home some snacks that are on offer downstairs at a small stall at the restaurant's entranceway.

There's not much more to say except, all round, it's a pleasant and worthwhile dining experience, especially for the price.

Ka Ka Lok Fast Food Chinese

G/F, 16 Ashley Road,
Tsim Sha Tsui

Hours:
8am-3am daily

2376 1198

Takeaway: Yes
Credit Cards: None

This place is quite unique and cheap, cheap, cheap. It's a fast-food takeaway-only place that offers nearly all its food for under $30.

Sandwiches, for example chicken and lettuce, are $8; rice and spaghetti dishes, for example, beef with either rice or spaghetti, are $20; and steak and chips is $21.50. Neither hamburgers nor fish and chips will break any banks at $6.50 and $14 respectively.

Sure, there's not much to it - the shop-front is open to the street and you share all the condiments at the front counter. Although the food quality is not fantastic, if it's a cheap meal you're after, then you can't beat Ka Ka Lok Fast Food.

Chinese

Kam Chiu Restaurant

Hours:
Open 24 hours

G/F, 56 Cameron Road,
Tsim Sha Tsui

Takeaway: Yes
Credit Cards: None

2366 6636

Located on busy Cameron Road, the Kam Chiu can be described as a Chinese restaurant with a try-hard Western style menu. Good or bad or middling, as the case is here, the restaurant offers two draw cards - one, cheap food and two, it's open 24 hours.

There's plenty on the menu with most dishes priced in the mid $30s. One of the set dinners, displayed proudly out the front of the restaurant in plastic, includes sirloin steak and vegetables, soup, a bun and a drink, all for $38.

Kam Chiu makes it into this guide more as a late night alternative than anything else; don't come here expecting the best quality food and you won't be disappointed.

Khyber Pass   Indian

Block E, 7/F, E-2,
Chungking Mansions,
36-44 Nathan Road,
Tsim Sha Tsui

2721 2786

Hours:
6pm-12am daily

Takeaway: Yes
Credit Cards: None

To get to the Khyber Pass restaurant you must first experience the ground floor lobby, the lift and then the seventh floor of the infamous Chungking Mansions (aka Little India or Pakistan). If that hasn't put you off, you'll find yourself in the right place for some cheap and good Indian food.

There's no beer on the menu but it will magically materialise if you ask for it. The vegetable curry for $30 is cheap and tasty, and the chicken vindaloo is perfect for hot-food lovers at $39. The sheek kebab ($48) makes a good starter and the naan ($8) comes authentically shaped as the tandoor.

Don't be surprised if the person sitting next to you is eating with their hands or if the other patrons appear mesmerised by the Bollywood songs playing on the TV - it all adds to the experience. Come to the Khyber Pass for really good, cheap food and to feel like you're in India for an hour or two.

Kung Tak Lam

Hours:
11am-11pm daily

1/F,
45-47 Carnarvon Road,
Tsim Sha Tsui

Takeaway: Yes
Credit Cards: V,MC,AE

2367 7881

With a branch also in Causeway Bay (see the Branches section for details), Kung Tam Lam is a welcome non-meat dining alternative in this meat-filled city.

Not only does it offer all-vegetarian meals but the vegetables are also organic and cooked with no MSG. For meat lovers or vegetarians who like to pretend they are eating meat, Kung Tam Lam offers a range of faux meat dishes, for example, the vegetarian goose ($48) which is basically all tofu. Nearly all the meals on the menu are between $48 and $58, which are not bad prices for a dose of health and a wide selection of vegetables (compared to the usual Hong Kong 'standard' when it comes to vegetables - choi sum).

Overall, the restaurant rates 'average' for the food but the staff are friendly.

Mabuhay   Filipino

11 Minden Avenue,   **Hours:**
Tsim Sha Tsui   9.30am-11pm daily

                                       Takeaway: Yes
2367 3762   **Credit Cards:** None

Filipinos are renowned for their hospitality and
love of music, and Mabuhay, with its Philippine
cuisine, friendly staff and romantic love songs, is
no exception. In operation for more than 20
years and frequented predominantly by Filipinos,
the menu is split into a few different sections,
including appetizers, native soups, Filipino dishes,
grilled and fried specialities, noodles and rice, and
Spanish dishes.

It's worth trying a few Filipino dishes because
there are not too many places in Hong Kong
where you get to sample this style of cooking
(unless you have a Filipina domestic helper, of
course). For example, there's the adobong pusit
(squid cooked with garlic, onions, tomatoes and
red pepper) for $40, and manok sa gata (chicken
in coconut milk gravy) for $45.

Prices are reasonable - most items are under $60
each - so drop in for a taste of Boracay or Cebu
(but just not on a Sunday when the place is
overrun by natives).

Macanese   **Macau Restaurant**

Hours:
6.30am-2.30am daily

25 Lock Road,
Tsim Sha Tsui

Takeaway: Yes
Credit Cards: None

2366 8148

If you are visiting Hong Kong, or if you are a lover of Macanese food, yet don't have time to get to Macau, then the Macau Restaurant will satisfy your desire to experience the traditional cuisine of the other SAR.

There are three branches in T.S.T. (see the Branches section for details) to choose from and another, aptly, in the Macau Ferry Terminal building in Sheung Wan (Shop 270-275, Shun Tak Shopping Centre, 2857 1933). The restaurant is open very early until very late and offers a range of 'chef-recommended' dishes such as: the Portuguese smoked duck breast for $38; the braised lamb knee for $58; and the baked cod fish with rice for $48. There's also Portuguese baked seafood rice for $58 and curry chicken for $48.

For a snack, or to finish off your meal, you must try the delicious Portuguese egg tart for $6.

Mall Cafe   International

YMCA,
41 Salisbury Road,
Tsim Sha Tsui

Hours:
7am-11.45pm daily

2268 7000

Takeaway: Yes
Credit Cards: V,MC,AE

Serving mainly YMCA hotel guests and members,
the Mall Café is also open to the public. The café
is typical of youth hostels around the world in that
it offers cheap food in a canteen style
atmosphere.

Breakfast is served from 7am to 11am as set
meals that include, depending on the type, fruit
juice, eggs, cereal, toast, pancakes or congee, for
up to $50. From 11am to closing time, there are
sandwiches, baked potatoes, pasta, more 'main'
meals and vegetarian dishes available that range
from $22 up to $60. There are also set lunches
and dinners (at set times) that include the choice
of a main dish and dessert and a drink for $54
and $70 respectively.

While the food isn't five-star, it's good value and
served in a wholesome environment.

Cafe   **Shadowman Cyber Cafe**

Hours: G/F, 7 Lock Road,
M to Sa: 8am-12am   **Tsim Sha Tsui**
Su: 9am-12am

Takeaway: Yes
Credit Cards: None   2366 5262

Tsim Sha Tsui

As the name suggests, the Shadowman Cyber Café is first and foremost an Internet access outlet but secondly, a café that intriguingly offers Halal food.

The deal is that with any purchase of food or drink, you get 20 minutes free internet usage which is then $10 thereafter for each 15 minutes, or without purchasing any food or drink you can pay $15 for the first 15 minutes or less and then $10 thereafter for each 15 minutes.

But now to the reason for its entry into this guidebook - the food. There are sandwiches on offer, mostly served in pita bread, for $35 to $48; beef or vegetable lasagne is $38; a beef burger is $32; and tandoori chicken is $30. There's also coffee, tea, drinks, desserts and other meals available.

Neither the food nor the Internet deal is bad, and the location is convenient, so log into this café especially if Halal food interests you.

Singapore Home Make   Singaporean

Shop D, G/F,
Hart Avenue Court,
19-23 Hart Avenue,
Tsim Sha Tsui

2368 8706

Hours:
11:30am-11pm daily

Takeaway: Yes
Credit Cards: V,MC,D

Some may know this restaurant as Singapore
Mrs. Chan Curry, but either way the Singapore
Home Make Restaurant offers dishes more
reminiscent of Singapore than Hong Kong.

These include satays (chicken, beef, pork and
lamb) for $48, and curries with rice, including
curry fish fillet served with rice, for $28. Noodles
and sandwiches are also on offer, as well as
chicken, vegetable and rice dishes, for fairly
decent prices.

In general, the food is average but the
environment is good. Seating is in booths, the
décor is trendy brown, and you can watch the
chef do his business in the window.

Come here for a taste of Singapore but at Hong
Kong prices.

Taiwan Chicken Farm

Hours:
11am-12am daily

78-80 Canton Road,
Tsim Sha Tsui

Takeaway: Yes
Credit Cards: V,MC,AE

2926 3088

Just next to the Happy Garden restaurant (also reviewed) are the two-in-one Taiwan Chicken Farm and Taiwan Beef Noodle restaurants. From the outside they appear to be separate but in fact they are one. Whatever the logic behind it, this is a good place to come to sample traditional Taiwanese fare.

Food prices are generally in the high $40s or above and the menus are split by restaurant. As a sample of the food and prices for the Taiwan Chicken Farm: BBQ pork with honey is $45; vegetables with salted duck's eggs and preserved duck's egg is $48; and fried boneless chicken with lemon sauce is $55. The Taiwan Beef Noodle restaurant offers fried mixed vegetables Taiwanese style for $55; noodles for $28 to $30; and Taiwanese snacks including sea blubber with chili for $35.

If this all sounds confusing and tempting, then go see and figure for yourself.

Thai & Vietnam   Thai / Vietnamese

G/F, Shop A,
Wardley Centre,
9-11 Prat Avenue,
Tsim Sha Tsui

2368 6181

Hours:
12pm-1am daily

Takeaway: Yes
Credit Cards: None

This light and bright little restaurant is a good find. If the retro looking plastic crockery doesn't capture your attention, then the fragrant aroma billowing from the kitchen certainly will.

The menu appears to be a little more Thai focused than Vietnamese and includes soup noodles for $28, rice noodles for $38 and curries for $48. The all-famous tom yum goong is $48 for a small or $68 for a larger size.

All in all, the Thai & Vietnam Restaurant exudes everything you love about South East Asia - tasty, good-value food using fresh produce, and that indelible service with a smile.

Food Hall — **The Cooked Deli**

Hours:
10.30am-10pm daily

Takeaway: Yes
Credit Cards: V,MC,AE,D

Basement,
Silvercord Building,
30 Canton Road,
Tsim Sha Tsui

2272 0812

The Cooked Deli in T.S.T. is generally the same as the one in Causeway Bay but with different food to choose from. The Food Hall set-up is similar and it also offers the Pit In - a convenience store cum mini supermarket and deli.

The Cooked Deli is a good place to come for various types of cuisine all under the one roof. As a sample of the selection, there's Anytime Now offering Asian rice and noodle dishes, including Indian chicken curry at $45; Sario, offering Chinese cuisine including dim sum at an average price of $15 for three pieces; and Figaro, serving Italian and European dishes, including a choice of pasta for $35 and pizzas at $28. There are also plenty of Japanese outlets, a well-known Honeymoon Chinese dessert bar, a Korean restaurant and other Chinese outlets too.

For a wide choice of cuisines and dishes, at reasonable prices and in a no-smoking environment, this is the place to come.

New Territories

The key centres of Sai Kung, Sha Tin, Tai Mei Tuk and Tai Po in the New Territories all offer a wide selection of budget eateries. So whether you live there, are visiting relatives or friends, or perhaps travelling through before or after a hike, you'll be pleased to know that economical dining possibilities await.

Sai Kung is known for its seafood and is a great place to eat and relax in after a hike in the neighbouring country parks. Sha Tin is the home of the New Town Plaza – a shopper's haven – as well as a range of restaurants. Tai Po itself has a number of different restaurants to choose from, as does the nearby village of Tai Mei Tuk where a restaurant scene has developed to satisfy hungry day-trippers.

Honeymoon Dessert Bar   Desserts

G/F, 10A Po Tung Road,
Sai Kung

Hours:
1:30pm-3am daily

2792 8533

Takeaway: Yes
Credit Cards: None

After you've eaten at one of the many restaurants in Sai Kung, why not top it all off with a treat from this locally famous dessert bar.

Although not located in the most salubrious of surroundings (it's right on the main road), the delicious food should take your mind off this fact.

You can choose from a huge range of desserts, for example, mango jelly for $22, red bean soup for $11 and papaya sago for $18.

And if you're craving something a little Western, then the banana pancake for $16 should satisfy you.

Indian

Indian Curry Hut

Hours:
11:30am-11:30pm daily

G/F, 64 Po Tung Road,
Sai Kung

Takeaway: Yes
Credit Cards: V,MC

2791 2929

The first thing that catches your eye about this restaurant is the small sign in the front window that reads 'No Smoking Seating Unavailable'.

The second thing is that the menu boasts free beer with the set meal.

Sitting on wooden table and chairs in a dimly lit room, listening to piped Indian music, you can enjoy a range of Indian favourites. From the tandoor, the chicken tikka is $52 and the sheek kebab is $56. Chicken and beef dishes, for example, chicken tikka masala and the beef vindaloo, are around the $52 mark.

Vegetarians are catered for too: a vegetable curry and the aloo gobi are both $46.

Kitaro   Japanese

G/F, 9A Po Tung Road,
Sai Kung

Hours:
M to F: 12pm-3pm
& 5:30pm-1am
Sa, Su & PH: 12pm-1am
Takeaway: Yes
Credit Cards: V,MC

2792 1423

Just near the Honeymoon Dessert Bar (also reviewed), the well-thumbed-at-the-edges menu signifies the popularity of this Japanese restaurant. The menu is traditional, as is the décor and lighting inside the restaurant.

As a sample of some of the cheaper meals available here: the Japanese roast pork udon noodles is $38; rice dishes, such as the chicken or pork cutlet and egg on rice are available for $40; and the assorted vegetable noodles soup is also $40.

The food servings are of a decent size and the waiter service is good.

For a variety of traditional Japanese food that is up to standard, the Kitaro Japanese Restaurant is recommended.

Thai   **Mai Thai Restaurant**

Hours: 32 Man Nin Street,
12pm-3pm   **Sai Kung**
& 6pm-11pm daily

Takeaway: Yes
Credit Cards: V,MC,D   2194 4553

Sai Kung is blessed with a few Thai restaurants
but this is the most modern and authentic.

The menu is eye-catchingly red and the listed
dishes are also written in Thai script.

The food is impressive. The tom yum kung
(soup) is $38 for a small size (you can also
choose medium and large), and the red prawn
curry is $58. Sweet and sour pork, beef or
chicken is one of the restaurant's favourites and is
available for $40. The Thai classic, pad Thai, is
$38.

For Thai food that is not so Chinese-influenced,
and not too badly priced, this is the place to
come.

Man Kee Thai   Thai

G/F, 65-67 Man Nin
Street,
Sai Kung

2791 9220

Sai Kung

This restaurant passes the basic 'Thai test'
because it displays a picture of the King and
Queen of Thailand in a prominent position.
However, whether the food itself passes the test is
debatable as it appears, in both taste and
presentation, to be quite Chinese-influenced.

Generally all food prices are $40 or more but, if
you come at lunchtime, there is a very good value
for money set menu available for $32. As an
example of some of the standard offerings and
prices: fried squid with chili and salt, and the
green curry chicken are both $48; and the mixed
vegetable with curry dish is $42.

Servings are large at this popular local restaurant.

If you like Chinese and/or Thai food, in large
amounts, then this place is worth a try, especially
at lunchtime when prices are cheaper.

Cafe **Pan Da Cafe**

Hours:
M: Closed
12pm-10pm daily

G/F, 23 See Cheung St.,
Sai Kung

Takeaway: Yes
Credit Cards: None

2791 6801

If you need a caffeine fix, this is the place for you. The small café, located one street back from the waterfront at the southern end of town, offers thirty types of coffee and more than ten different kinds of tea. For an expresso, expect to pay $15, for a mocha - $30, and $60 for a cup of Jamaican Blue Mountain coffee. Strawberry or apple tea costs $25.

There is also food available here that can be eaten either outside on a small raised terrace overlooking the little street, or inside below walls lined with pictures of vegetables and fruit. Pasta dishes, for example, spaghetti bolognaise, are $48; rice dishes are similarly priced; sandwiches and toasties range from $22 to $30; and salads go up to $35 for a smoked salmon dish.

This is a nice place to sit on a sunny day while indulging in a dose of caffeine.

Ryo Zan Paku

Japanese

G/F, 54 Po Tung Road,
Sai Kung

Hours:
12pm-3pm
& 6pm-12am daily

Takeaway: Yes
Credit Cards: V,MC

2791 1030

Just along from the Indian Curry Hut, the Ryo Zan Paku Japanese Restaurant offers traditional Japanese food to famous and not-so-famous diners alike.

Meals include sushi, ramen, sashimi and grilled dishes such as lamb and eel. For a sample of some of the cheaper meals on offer: the seafood noodles/udon is $48; the roast chicken rice box is $55; and the ramen lunch sets - including beef, pork, seafood and mixed vegetables - are good value at $35.

The environment is quite comfortable but the lighting is a little dim.

All in all, a good place to come if you want to see or be seen and experience decent Japanese food.

Bar / Cafe

Steamers Bar

Hours:
9am-12am daily

23 Chan Man Street,
Sai Kung

Takeaway: Yes
Credit Cards: V,MC,AE,D

2792 6991

This place is called a 'bar' but it has a 'café' feel about it as well, especially during the daytime.

Following the local nautical theme, the walls are blue and the wood décor of the restaurant and bar is a classic soft beige hue.

The meals are very typical café/bar. A steak sandwich will set you back $55, and a veggi melt is $45. For more main meals, you can get a vegetable lasagne for $50 and bangers and mash for $55.

If you're looking for somewhere to have breakfast in Sai Kung, then you're well catered for here - for example, you can get an omelette for $48.

For a change from Asian cuisine, this place is not a bad choice for reasonably priced meals.

Thai Beach Restaurant   Thai

Shop 1 & 2, G/F,
Siu Yat House,
Hoi Pong Square,
Sai Kung

2791 1561

Hours:
11am-12am daily

Takeaway: Yes
Credit Cards: None

The Thai Beach Restaurant wouldn't look out of place on Koh Samui or Koh Samet in Thailand. It tries to look like a bamboo hut and is located in a great spot to catch the breeze from the sea.

It has an extensive menu offering the usual Thai fare. The curries range from $48 to $58 and include roast duck, chicken, pork, beef, vegetables and even prawns.

Charcoal grilled squid is $48; tom yum kung is $38 for a small; and the fried morning glory with crispy pork is $42.

Come here for the 'nearly' seafront location and down-to-earth Thai food with a beach-like feel.

Chinese

King Lam Kok

Hours:
M to F: 11am-2:30pm
& 5:30pm-11pm
Sa & Su: 11am-11pm
Takeaway: Yes
Credit Cards: V,MC

Shop 169-170, Phase 1,
New Town Plaza,
Sha Tin

2602 2595

King Lam Kok has no English writing to announce its name so look for the long restaurant with green seats at the end of the Level 1 food court area.

The restaurant, owned by a friendly Chinese/ Australian, offers local fare including: braised fish in chili sauce for $60; diced chicken with cashew nuts for $58; and cold souped sliced beef for $45.

With most pork and beef dishes generally priced up to $55, King Lam Kok is one of the cheaper restaurants located in the New Town Plaza.

Sha Tin

Yukiguni Ramen

Japanese

Shop 140-151, Phase 1,
New Town Plaza,
Sha Tin

Hours:
11am-10:30pm daily

2696 9708

Takeaway: Yes
Credit Cards: V,MC,D

The Yukiguni Ramen restaurant looks quite inviting from the outside, with fake food and a not-too-big menu displayed. However, inside, the seats are quite close together, and the food and service are average.

Nevertheless, there are not too many other cheap restaurants to choose from in this neck of the woods, so if you feel like Japanese then you can try: ramens, including chicken wing dumpling ramen, ranging from $38 to $54; or rice dishes, including the teriyaki pork with rice, for $48.

There's also an a-la-carte menu that includes chicken wings for $40 and salmon sashimi for $60.

Don't go out of your way to come here, and don't expect too much when you arrive, and you won't be too disappointed.

Thai   **Chili Chili**

Hours:
M to F: 11am-11pm
Sa: 7:30pm-2am
Su: 7:30am-11pm
Takeaway: Yes
Credit Cards: V,MC

G/F, 101 Lung Mei
Village, Ting Kok Road,
Tai Po

2662 6767

Tai Mei Tuk

Located at the end of the restaurant strip (or the
start, depending on how you look at it), Chili Chili
is the newest and most modern restaurant in the
area. The outside wooden seating with umbrellas
overlooks the bike path, then the road, with
glimpses of Tolo Harbour and further views of the
mountains.

The menu includes a range of cuisines but most
notably Thai and Cantonese. The Guangdong
specials range from $58 to $68 and include the
tasty-sounding deep fried fish with salt and chili,
sautéed shrimps with nuts and sweet corn, and
the sautéed beef tenderloin with pineapple. The
curries - green and red - are $52, which is a little
more expensive than other Thai restaurants
nearby. Noodles start at $30 and the chef's
specials are around the $60 mark.

This place certainly has potential - the décor and
location are a cut above the other restaurants and
the food is satisfactory and nicely presented.

Chung Shing Thai

G/F, 69 Tai Mei Tuk
Village, Ting Kok Road,
Tai Po

2664 5218

Hours:
M to Sa: 12pm-3pm
& 6pm-12am
Su: 6pm-12am
Takeaway: Yes
Credit Cards: None

Tai Mei Tuk

Connected organisationally to the Chinese restaurant of the same name, the Chung Shing Thai Restaurant gets good reviews all round.

It is not easy to locate as signage, in English at least, is scarce so look for the restaurant next to Wong's and you'll be there. Like all the restaurants in the strip, the seating is outside but under cover; however, unlike the others, this place is nearly always full.

The restaurant offers not only Thai food but also local fare. Curries - green or red and with beef, pork or chicken - start at $45; pork chop with lemongrass flavours goes for $50; and seafood fried rice in a pineapple is $60. The Chinese food on offer goes cheaply for $40 or less.

It's recommended that you come here with a group so that you can try a range of the delicious dishes.

Chung Shing Traditional

Hours:
M to F: 12pm-10pm
Sa & Su: 11am-11pm

G/F, 36B Tai Mei Tuk
Village, Ting Kok Road,
Tai Po

Takeaway: Yes
Credit Cards: None

2662 6162

Tai Mei Tuk

The Chung Shing Traditional Restaurant is renowned as being one of, if not 'the', original founders of the restaurant scene in Tai Mei Tuk.

Located just off the main strip, the restaurant offers customary local food served at standard large round tables, with mini BBQs atop, in an outside seating environment. The seafood is generally expensive but the other dishes are reasonably priced. These include: fried pork chop with special sauces for $45; fried boneless chicken in lemon sauce for $58; and a vegetable vermicelli hot pot for $48. The cheapest seafood is fried squid with chilli pepper for $55.

The food is satisfactory and the service is worth a note, proven by the considerable number of patrons at any mealtime.

Mali-bu Thai

G/F, 27A Lung Mei
Village, Ting Kok Road,
Tai Po

Hours:
11:30am-12am daily

Takeaway: Yes
Credit Cards: V,MC,D

2948 2802

The Mali-bu Thai Cuisine restaurant is popular with locals and foreigners alike and enjoys good reviews from all. It's lit up like a Christmas tree and plays Western style music at night, but with a traditional Thai feel. There are statues of Thai women at the door and pictures of the King and Queen of the Kingdom adorn the rear wall.

As well as the atmosphere, the food and service can be described as above standard. Noodle dishes start at $32 and the tasty main dishes start at $42, including: sweet curry beef and red or green curry chicken from $45; baked seafood rice in pineapple for $58; and fried mussels with garlic for $50.

As a special mention, the fish is very fresh but is generally a little expensive, and the tom yam kung is tasty and not too hot.

Pinocchio Garden

Hours:
11am-1am daily

G/F, 60 Lung Mei
Village, Ting Kok Road,
Tai Po

Takeaway: No
Credit Cards: V,MC

2662 5826

Tai Mei Tuk

The Pinocchio Garden Restaurant is located just off the main eating strip - look for the gaudy 'I love you' neon sign and you'll find it.

The main thing different about this restaurant, compared to others in the area, is that it offers Portuguese food and wine. It also offers an extensive menu, including Thai food. Some of the choices on offer include: charcoal broiled Portuguese sausage for $30; sweet and sour chicken for $48; and the pork chop (baked with cheese) for $50. The Thai curries range in price from $40 to $65; and noodle, rice and spaghetti dishes start at $38.

If you feel like some non-Asian food then this is really the only place to visit in Tai Mei Tuk.

Wong's

G/F, 69A Tai Mei Tuk
Village,
Tai Po

Hours:
11:00am-10:30pm daily

2948 2282

Takeaway: Yes
Credit Cards: V,MC

Wong's Restaurant has a fast food feel to it,
mainly due to the colourful backlit pictures of food
that line the roof. But it's not a fast food
restaurant and patrons enjoy their time reading
the complimentary magazines and eating the
large range of Chinese dishes.

Traditional hotpots are a speciality and include the
seafood and mixed vegetable hotpot, and the
curry beef brisket hotpot, for $55 each. The BBQ
and soy dishes start at $45 and include pigeon in
soy sauce, and honey BBQ pork, for $48. There
are other seafood dishes also available that won't
break the bank; for example, the baked garoupa
fillet in cheese and butter sauce for $60. Then
there are vegetable, poultry and pork dishes
starting at $40, and rice and noodle dishes for an
average of $30.

Overall, Wong's is a friendly place that has plenty
of decent food on offer at reasonable prices.

Indian   **Cosmopolitan Curry House**

Hours:
11.30am-12am daily

80 Kwong Fuk Road,
Tai Po

Takeaway: Yes
Credit Cards: V,MC

2658 6915

The Cosmopolitan Curry House is an institution in Tai Po - especially famous for its curries. There is a huge menu on offer and most meals are served with rice or naan bread.

All the Indian favourites are available. Mutton and chicken dishes, including the mutton madras and madras chicken curry, are $55; vegetable dishes are $40; fish dishes range from $49 to $64; and beef dishes, including beef vindaloo, range from $49 to $56. To sample the famous curries, a curry set dinner is also available that includes cream soup or Russian borsch, a curry, chapatti or rice, and a drink. The prices for the set meals vary depending on the choice of curry - for example, the peach fish curry 'meal deal' is $61 and the East Indies curry set meal is $59.

The Cosmopolitan Curry House is definitely worth a visit if you're in town; even if you are from 'out of town', the journey will certainly be worth it.

Little Egret

Tai Po Kau Village,
4339 Tai Po Road,
Tai Po

2657 6628

Hours:
11am-11pm daily

Takeaway: Yes
Credit Cards: V,MC

Tai Po

You may have wondered about this large, pinkish-coloured, Mediterranean-style building with a small lake out the front, which can be seen from the KCR train before you approach Tai Po Market station. Well, it's the Tai Po Kau Interactive Nature Centre and inside is not only the Museum of Ethnology but also the Little Egret Restaurant.

While the décor in the restaurant is quite pleasant and different, the food can really only be described as 'so-so'. The prices are at the higher end of the cheap scale and include the baked seafood fried rice, and the baked pork chop fried rice, both for $60. Chicken tagliolini and quesadilla are examples of the other fare available, but are priced in the $70s.

Don't be surprised to see some 'signature' small egrets wandering around the lake area while you are eating your meal or having a post-meal walk.

Indian

Shalimar Indian

Hours:
11.30am-3pm
& 6pm-11pm daily

G/F, 127 Kwong Fuk
Road,
Tai Po

Takeaway: Yes
Credit Cards: V,MC,AE

2653 7790

As one would expect, Shalimar Indian Restaurant offers all things Indian - that is, decent Indian food, Indian paintings that adorn the walls, and Indian staff who serve the food and your needs well.

There's quite a selection of food to choose from, served with rice or naan bread, including: rogan josh or beef korma for $58; chicken tikka for $52; and the vegetable kebab from the tandoor for $50. There are also relatively cheap lunch sets available that come with rice or naan bread - for example, the curry chicken lunch set for $30.

All in all this is not a bad place to come, especially for the cheaper lunchtime meals, if you happen to be in Tai Po.

Outlying Islands

Tripping out to one of Hong Kong's outlying islands need not involve taking a picnic basket. The islands of Cheung Chau, Lamma, Lantau and Peng Chau all offer a good range of eateries that are not expensive.

Cheung Chau's waterfront is a great place to watch the sun go down over the fishing boats in the harbour while eating the day's fresh catch. On Lamma Island, most of the cheaper restaurants are located at Yung Shue Wan where the cuisines are diverse, influenced by a large expatriate population. Lantau Island offers not only hiking, swimming and tourist attractions but also a wide range of eateries and cuisines, particularly in the main areas of Mui Wo, Cheung Sha, Discovery Bay and Ngong Ping. And then there's Peng Chau which, for a small island, also offers a few eating possibilities.

Bayview

Cafe

Warwick Hotel,
East Bay,
Cheung Chau

Hours:
8am-6pm daily

2981 0081

Takeaway: Yes
Credit Cards: V,MC,AE,D

Located inside the Warwick Hotel, with views over the sea, this snack café is suited more to holidaymakers or residents of the hotel. But the general public is welcome and it's not a bad place to escape the summer heat while retaining the views over Tung Wan Beach.

The menu is only snacks, so don't come here expecting anything too substantial. As an example of the snack fare: a hamburger on a bun is $45; fish and chips are $40; and the Warwick clubhouse sandwich is $50.

The enclosed seating is ideal for hungry beachgoers who want to take a break from the heat.

Chinese   **East Lake Restaurant**

Hours: G/F, 85 Tung Wan Road,
10am-10pm daily   **Cheung Chau**

Takeaway: Yes
Credit Cards: None   2981 3869

The East Lake Restaurant is recommended for a
few reasons. One is that it is located near to Tung
Wan Beach - meaning you can enjoy the sand and
sea and then not have to walk too far for a meal.

Secondly, the staff are friendly and efficient.

Thirdly, the food is reasonably priced and,
fourthly, it doesn't taste too bad either. As an
example, you can get the grilled duck (half) with
lemon for $50; fried beef and cashew nuts for
$48; or sweet and sour pork with vegetables for
$45. Also, the fried mixed vegetables are $40
and the deep fried squid is $48.

Lastly, and uniquely, you can even buy your own
seafood from the nearby seafront fish markets
and then ask the chef to cook it for you.

Long Island Restaurant Chinese

G/F,
51-53 San Hing Street,
Cheung Chau

2981 1678

Cheung Chau

To sum it up, in their own words, the Long Island Restaurant offers 'over 100 varieties of traditional dim sum with different typical style' and 'traditional Chinese food and seafood inside and outside'.

As a sample of the menu and prices: fish head in soup is $38; spiced salt frogs are $48; and steamed pigeon with dried lily flower, black fungus and lotus leaf is $38. Seafood claypots and vegetable dishes, for example, the exotic-sounding eight treasures pot, average $48 in price.

Located on the main harbour strip, this is the place to come to experience Chinese fare in all its different forms.

Indian   **Morocco's**

Hours: G/F,
4pm-3am daily   71 San Hing Street,
                                  Cheung Chau

Takeaway: Yes
Credit Cards: None   2986 9767

With some outside seating on a raised deck and
located only 100 metres from the ferry pier, this
is a good place for people-watching and enjoying
a cuisine that differs to the rest of the Cheung
Chau fare.

The staff are friendly and the food's not bad. The
fish kadai ($60) is tasty, so too are the samosas
($25) and the chicken tikka ($50). There are
plenty more traditional Indian dishes to choose
from, mostly around the $50 to $60 mark.

While this restaurant has an Indian feel due to the
food, the music and the videos playing, it also has
a decidedly local feel with a darts board and
cartoon pictures of local restaurant enthusiasts
lining the walls.

New Baccarat

9A Pak She Praya Road,
Cheung Chau

Hours:
11:30am-11pm daily

2981 0606

Takeaway: Yes
Credit Cards: V,MC

The New Baccarat Restaurant (look for blue checks on the tablecloths) is found at the end of the row of seafront eateries, furthest from the pier.

It offers one of the cheapest seafood menus around, including: fried shrimps with vegetables ($55); baked garoupa with cheese and butter ($55); sweet and sour prawns in pineapple ($58); and fried squid with minced garlic ($45). For non-fish eaters, there is also a range of poultry, hotpots, pork, beef and vegetable dishes available from $45 to $55, or rice and noodle dishes from $25 to $45.

Come here to enjoy the sunset and a selection of seafood, at reasonable prices, in a relaxed atmosphere.

Chinese   **Sea Dragon King**

Hours: Corner of Praya Street
10am-11:30pm daily   and Tai Hing Tai Road,
                                   Cheung Chau

Takeaway: Yes
Credit Cards: None   2981 1699

Not unlike the other open-air restaurants lining
the harbour, the Sea Dragon King Restaurant
offers the standard Cheung Chau seafood
bonanza. You can choose from the restaurant's
great display of fruits-of-the-sea but be warned
these fish don't come too cheaply.

There is a simple menu, however, that offers a
fresh and tasty sample of the sea at reasonable
prices. For example, the fried shrimp with cashew
nuts is $60; the fried squid with salt and pepper is
$54; and the fried squid with broccoli is $47.
Besides seafood, you can also opt for local style
pork, beef, chicken and vegetable dishes that
range in price up to $47.

The atmosphere at this restaurant is similar to the
others nearby, but a little bit simpler, which
certainly does not detract from the fresh taste of
the seafood.

The Garden

Pub

Tung Wan Road,
Cheung Chau

2981 4610

Takeaway: No
Credit Cards: None

This place is renowned for being the oldest café/pub serving Western style food on Cheung Chau.

It's mainly a haunt for drinkers so the food menu is quite limited, but it's cheap.

You can order the usual pub-like fare of French fries for $20; burgers for $30 to $45; onion rings for $35; and sandwiches for $35 to $40. There are a few different fillings you can choose from for the burgers and sandwiches, which accounts for the range in prices.

All this can be washed down with your favourite pint of beer - or shot of tequila - or other beverage.

International   **Arroy Thai**

Hours: 67 Main Street,
8am-10:30pm daily   Yung Shue Wan,
                                          Lamma Island

Takeaway: Yes
Credit Cards: None   2982 1150

Even though Arroy Thai offers some Thai dishes,
don't go there expecting authentic Thai cuisine.

The Thai food - eight, mainly curry, dishes
ranging in price from $35 to $45 - is served from
a hot bain marie, is not offered on Fridays, and
the authenticity of the ingredients is questionable.

Really, Arroy Thai offers a mixed bag of cheap
and filling non-Thai food. Pizzas range from $30
to $48; sandwiches range from $15 to $26; and
there's a large breakfast menu, served from 8am
to 3pm, that includes pancakes for $16.

The restaurant is very casual and you can sit
inside, at the bar, or out at the street-side tables.

B&B

International

22 Main Street,
Yung Shue Wan,
Lamma Island

2982 4388

Hours:
M to F: 12pm–12am
Sa, Su & PH: 12pm-2am

Takeaway: Yes
Credit Cards: V,MC,AE

Just near Blue Bird (also reviewed), and underneath Yung Shue Wan's banyan tree, is the B&B restaurant. This place is a bit 'hit and miss' in terms of food quality, but it's known for its friendly and hospitable staff.

With wine displayed out the front, the main courses are quite pricey at over $100 each. There are some cheaper dishes, however: the spaghetti and rice dishes are around $58, which include spaghetti bolognaise and seafood fried rice; and there are salads and sandwiches available that range from $38 for a tuna fish salad to $58 for a green salad.

While the range of cheaper meals on offer is limited, the outdoor seating overlooking the sea is certainly a bonus.

Japanese   **Blue Bird**

Hours:
11:30am-1am daily

G/F, 24 Main Street,
Yung Shue Wan,
Lamma Island

Takeaway: No
Credit Cards: None

2982 0687

The Blue Bird Japanese Restaurant has a good
reputation on Lamma and also at its other branch
on Ap Lei Chau (see the Branches section for
details).

It's recognised as having traditional food that
tastes good and is not too expensive. The
atmosphere is also quite traditional with wooden
chairs and tables and seating around a kitchen
bar inside. There's also appealing seating
outside, at the back of the restaurant, with views
over the sea to the Lamma pier. As a sample of
the food and its prices: from the teppanyaki bar,
sliced pork with ginger sauce is $35, and the king
prawn and U.S. beef dishes are both $55. Grilled
salmon is $45 and grilled squid with sauce is $35;
and tempura dishes range from $35 to $50. There
are also noodles, rice and hotpot dishes to choose
from to easily satisfy your taste buds.

If you like fine Japanese food at reasonable
prices, then Blue Bird is a must.

Bookworm Cafe

79 Main Street,
Yung Shue Wan,
Lamma Island

2982 4838

Hours:
M to F: 10am-7pm
Sa: 9am-11pm
Su: 9am-9pm
Takeaway: Yes
Credit Cards: V,MC

Lamma Island

Much has been written about the Bookworm Café and it's all good. This café is quite unique, not only for Lamma but also for Hong Kong, and is more reminiscent of the semi-hippy cafes you'd find in Western cities like Melbourne or Vancouver.

It offers vegetarian cuisine, organic health food and a focal point for community issues and interaction. The food is healthy and fresh. Breakfasts range from $20 for a bagel to $60 for a vegie omelette; the shepherdess pie (made from lentils and beans) and salad is $55; and Lebanese bread sandwiches are $25. The goat's cheese sanga is delicious at $45.

In line with its name and the atmosphere, you can read books and magazines from the shelves while dining, and purchase second-hand books as well.

Overall, this is a great place and is well worth a visit.

Concerto Inn

Hours:
8am-10pm daily

28 Hung Shing Ye Beach,
Yung Shue Wan,
Lamma Island

Takeaway: Yes
Credit Cards: V,MC,D

2982 1668

Lamma Island

Concerto Inn is one of the best-located 'inns' and restaurants on Lamma - it overlooks the popular Hung Shing Ye Beach (and the not-as-popular power station) and is only a five-minute walk from the main strip at Yung Shue Wan.

Going by Lamma standards, the food is a little pricey and is strangely priced with the inclusion of cents. For example, the chef-recommended nasi goreng is $56.80; the chicken satay is $48.80 and the clubhouse sandwich with French fries is $52.80. There are also salads, sandwiches, 'Asian favourites' and snacks to choose from, including French fries for $24.80.

The food is not the best around, the décor may be a bit cheesy (faux grass and plastic furniture) but you certainly can't beat the location.

Green Cottage

Cafe

G/F, 15A Main Street,
Yung Shue Wan,
Lamma Island

Hours:
M to F: 5:30am-5:30pm
Sa & Su: 7:30am-8:30pm

2982 6934

Takeaway: Yes
Credit Cards: None

Like the Bookworm Café (also reviewed), the Green Cottage offers vegetarian food and fruit smoothies but in a smaller, more hole-in-the-wall café style. It's quite rustic - you can sit on colourful seats, eat from upturned wooden wheels used as tables, and watch the ferry coming in and out.

There's not a huge range to choose from but you can have a vegetable pie for $25; croissants or muffins for $7; and fruit smoothies for $25.

The Green Cottage also sells a range of health food items for the more health-conscious patron.

This is a good little café to grab a healthy bite and drink at before catching the ferry.

International **Holiday Mood Grill**

Hours:
Tu: Closed
M to Su: 11am-10:30pm

Takeaway: Yes
Credit Cards: V,MC,D,AE

G/F, 26 Main Street,
Yung Shue Wan,
Lamma Island

2982 2328

Lamma Island

The Holiday Mood restaurant lives up to its name. If the chefs and waiters are in a good mood, a visit here will be satisfying; but if not, then the experience may be disappointing.

The restaurant offers a range of meals, most of which can be aptly described as 'attempted Western', and includes some Thai dishes. Offerings include the grilled salted pork fillet for $32 and the deep fried fish with chili sweet and sour sauce for $36.

A cake stall out the front might grab your attention, so too the seaview seating out the back.

Lamcombe Seafood   Chinese

G/F, 47 Main Street,
Yung Shue Wan,
Lamma Island

2982 0881

Hours:
10:30am-10:30pm daily

Takeaway: Yes
Credit Cards: V,MC,AE,D

There are plenty of choices for seafood on Lamma but the Lamcombe Seafood Restaurant is recommended in Yung Shue Wan.

Generally, the seafood is sold at market prices but there are some reasonably priced seafood meals available: for example, the sautéed fresh squid with green vegetable is $55, and the crab with fish soup is $60. There are plenty of non-seafood meals available too. The honeyed BBQ ribs and the pork chop with salad are both $60, and the rice and noodle dishes start at $38.

One of the best things about this restaurant is the environment - there's outdoor seating overlooking the small harbour out the back, away from the relative madness of the main street. The staff are very kid-friendly and provide great service.

Definitely a relaxing place to while away a lazy Sunday afternoon.

Chinese

Lung Kong

Hours:
8am-4am daily

G/F, 38 Main Street,
Yung Shue Wan,
Lamma Island

Takeaway: Yes
Credit Cards: None

2982 0025

Lung Kong is a very down-to-earth Chinese restaurant with Western food items also available (Chinese style, that is). It's cheap and cheerful, run by a friendly family, and has plenty of outdoor seating in its corner location.

The range of food to choose from includes: sweet and sour pork for $45; squid or mixed vegetables with curry sauce for $50; and noodles for $30. There's even some rarely-found 'cheapish' seafood, for example: curry prawns with rice for $45, or steamed mussels with garlic for $55. And the Western dishes include pork chops with vegetables and fried beef with pineapple, both for $55.

Don't come here expecting the finest of restaurants but you'll get a friendly feed nonetheless.

Pizza Milano Italian

Flat A, G/F & 1/F,
2 Back Street,
Yung Shue Wan,
Lamma Island

2982 4848

Hours:
M to F: 6pm-4am
Sa & Su: 2pm-12am

Takeaway: Yes
Credit Cards: None

Pizza Milano gets good reviews all round. The staff are friendly, there's al fresco seating available, the food is good (the pizza crust is 'just right') and it's reasonably priced.

There are a range of tasty pizza toppings and sizes to choose from. Small pizzas, with four slices, range from $50 to $70; and the regular and large pizzas, with six and eight slices respectively, are big enough to share (the pizza and the cost) and start from $62. The calzones also come recommended but are a little pricier at $87. And, being an Italian restaurant, there's also pasta, salad, lasagne, crostinis and snacks to tempt your taste buds.

If you can't get to Lamma but you still want to experience a Milano meal, then you'll be pleased to know that there is also a branch in Central (see the Branches section for details).

Sau Kee Seafood

Hours:
10:30am-10:30pm daily

43 Main Street,
Yung Shue Wan,
Lamma Island

Takeaway: Yes
Credit Cards: V,MC

2982 0210

Sau Kee Seafood Restaurant offers seafood and
Chinese meals to a more local clientele than
Lamcombe's more 'gweilo' crowd next door (also
reviewed). Sau Kee offers outside seating with
sea views, as well as inside seating in a light and
clean restaurant.

When it comes to the food, the prices are quite
satisfactory too. You can choose from deep fried
cuttlefish for $55; Singapore noodles for $35; and
fried pigeon for $60. There are also plenty of
seafood dishes on offer and, as per the standard,
their prices are market determined.

The harbour view seating out the back is definitely
a winner for this restaurant and, with big, round
tables, makes for good group dining.

Spicy Island

Indian

23 Main Street,
Yung Shue Wan,
Lamma Island

Hours:
12pm-12am daily

2982 0830

Takeaway: No
Credit Cards: None

The Spicy Island restaurant offers the greatest selection and most refined Indian food on Lamma. While most seating is inside, there's also some outdoor seating that allows you to soak up the relaxed Lamma atmosphere.

The prices aren't too bad either. The chicken and mutton specialities are almost all $50 and include such dishes as the chicken korma and the mutton vindaloo. The biryanis range from $40 upwards, and the large range of vegetarian specialities are mostly $40. The tandoori and seafood items are a little higher in price, but you can still taste these delights for $45 for the chicken tikka or $55 for the fish Goa curry.

If you are looking for authentic Indian food and you are already on Lamma, then this is the place to come.

Chinese   **Kung Shing**

Hours: G/F, 35 Lower Cheung
8am-9pm daily   Sha Village,
                                    Lantau Island

Takeaway: Yes
Credit Cards: None   2980 2711

If The Stoep (also reviewed) is full, as it often is,
or if you prefer Chinese food, then try the Kung
Shing Restaurant. Located next door, it enjoys
the same fine view of the sea and also has
outdoor seating with tables and chairs on the
beach.

The food here is standard Chinese fare with some
dishes that are more reminiscent of those found in
'Westernised' Chinese restaurants. For the main
course, sweet and sour pork with pineapple is
$45, fried squid with chilli and salt comes deep
fried at $50, and the BBQ fillet of pork is $60.
Rice dishes are around the $40 mark, including
sliced garoupa and vegetables on rice.
Vegetarian dishes are also available, ranging from
$30 for vegetables with oyster sauce to $60 for
vegetables with cashew nuts.

This is a great place if you're feeling homesick for
the Chinese food you get back home, and you
can't beat the location.

The Stoep

International

32 Lower Cheung Sha
Village,
Lantau Island

Hours:
Tu to Su: 12pm–10pm

2980 2699

Takeaway: No
Credit Cards: None

The Stoep is located right on the edge of one of
Hong Hong's best beaches. Open-air seating (with
some tables and chairs actually on the sand)
overlooks the beach, making this a favourite
restaurant among day and junk trippers and
locals alike.

Technically, the Stoep shouldn't make it into this
guide since the main meat meals - cooked on the
braai or BBQ - are generally over $100 each, but
it is possible to eat great food here for less. As a
sample of the menu: salads are available from
$25; grilled vegetables for $50; seafood soup is
$55; a range of extremely tasty dips, for example
hummus and tzatziki, are $25 per portion;
marinated salmon steak with mustard sauce is
$50; and the divine chorizo sausages and green
onions dish is $60.

A fantastic restaurant in a fantastic location that
always receives rave reviews, The Stoep is
definitely worth a visit.

Asian   **Chilli n' Spice**

Hours:
M to F: 11:30am-2:30pm
& 5:30pm-12am
Sa & Su: 11:30am-12pm
Takeaway: Yes
Credit Cards: V,MC,AE

Shop 102, 1/F,
Discovery Bay Plaza,
Discovery Bay,
Lantau Island

2987 9191

Chilli' n' Spice is mainly an Asian restaurant but
with an interesting addition of an Italian pizza
trade. The restaurant has the same layout and
great view as Jade Lotus (also reviewed), which is
located next door.

Green curry duck is served spicing hot for $55;
shredded beef with mango is $60; and fried rice
noodles Indonesian style is $48. For pizzas, you
can choose regular or large in size, and both work
out cheaper if shared. The toppings are
interesting and are a fusion with the restaurant's
other fare; for example, there's a Thai spicy
seafood pizza and a chilli con carne pizza.

The food quality is okay, the prices are okay and
both are topped off with a good view.

See the Branches section for details of sister
restaurants.

Ebeneezer's   International

Shop G06,
Discovery Bay Plaza,
Discovery Bay,
Lantau Island

2987 0036

Hours:
10am-12am daily

Takeaway: Yes
Credit Cards: None

Ebeneezer's bills itself as serving 'the most healthiest and delicious kebabs in Hong-Kong'. And they're not far wrong. The Lebanese pita bread and meat are 'just right' and taste even better after a choice of dressings is added.

Also with a branch in Wanchai (see the Branches section), Ebeneezer's is really a takeaway shop that also offers curries, pizzas, biryanis, salads, sandwiches and some 'special' meals like fish'n'chips and beef lasagne. Prices all round are reasonable: a regular kebab is $40 to $45, and the rest of the food offerings are all around $40. Pizzas, for example, the chicken tikka pizza, are around $60 for a regular or up to $95 for a large that could be shared.

This is first and foremost a kebab shop so stick to the main fare and you won't be disappointed.

Chinese   **Jade Lotus**

Hours:
11.30am-2.30pm
& 6pm-10.30pm daily

Takeaway: Yes
Credit Cards: V,MC

Shop 103, 1/F,
Discovery Bay Plaza,
Discovery Bay,
Lantau Island

2987 8033

Serving mainly traditional Peking, Shanghai and Sichuan dishes, this place is 'not bad' and has great views overlooking the beach.

As per usual, the seafood dishes are more expensive but there are also poultry, vegetable, beef, mutton, pork and noodles and rice dishes which are more reasonably priced. For example, the sweet and sour chicken is $55; fried noodles Shanghai style is $45; and ginger beef with chilli sauce is $60. The crispy rice dishes are recommended for their unique serving style (the rice and meat are served separately, and the meat is then poured over the top of the crispy rice making a tantalising sizzling sound) and delicious taste. For those taking-away, there's a separate outside window offering, amongst other things, the popular Chinese cured sausage with rice for $26.

For a taste of mainland cuisine with a nice view, this is a good place to come.

Jo Jo Indian

Indian

Shop 101, 1/F,
Discovery Bay Plaza,
Discovery Bay,
Lantau Island

2987 0122

Hours:
11am-3pm
& 6pm-11pm daily

Takeaway: Yes
Credit Cards: V,MC,D,AE

Jo Jo Indian Food doesn't offer the beach view that other restaurants in the vicinity do but the food comes recommended as 'worth a try'.

All the usual Indian dishes are on the menu served to your preference of hot, medium or mild. Most prices hover between the $60 to $70 mark (and more for seafood) but there are some for under $60. You can choose murgh tikka (chicken) from the tandoor for $58, and a range of vegetarian dishes for around $42. Jal frezi gosht (lamb) is $58, and there are soups for around $35.

Try it if you are looking for a change from the Northern or South East Asian fare that is mostly on offer in D.B.

Also see the Branches section for details of its sister restaurant in Tsuen Wan.

Chinese   **Sea Plaza Food Centre**

Hours:
10.30am-12am daily

Discovery Bay Plaza,
Discovery Bay,
Lantau Island

Takeaway: Yes
Credit Cards: None

This local 'dai pai dong' is huge and offers a vast array of fast-food meals for under $35.

You can choose from BBQ delights, Chinese food, Western dishes and South Asian style cuisine. As a sample from each menu category: red, green and yellow curries are $35; BBQ pork with curry rice is $32; fried noodles with BBQ pork are $35; and sliced beef with tomato rice (Western style) is $32.

While prices are a little high compared to other local eateries around Hong Kong, it's still the cheapest place to eat in Discovery Bay.

Shougon

Korean

Discovery Bay Plaza,
Discovery Bay,
Lantau Island

2987 6151

Hours:
M to F: 11.30am-2.30pm
& 5.30pm-10.30pm
Sa&Su: 11.30am-10.30pm
Takeaway: Yes
Credit Cards: V,MC,D,AE

With grill plates on each table, the BBQ dishes are the main reason to come here. Plus there's a great view over the beach if you sit near the window.

Overall though, the Korean dishes have a decidedly Hong Kong style and taste to them. Nevertheless, cooking the BBQ yourself at your table is a novelty and you can choose from pork, chicken, beef, fish and ox-tongue for around $55. The Korean stone pot rice (chicken, beef or clams) is $52 and pleasingly spicy. There are also noodle and soup sets to choose from where you can choose your ingredients, the soup base and the rice or noodle (for example, the spicy beef shank for $38).

Remember to get a seaview table here to enhance your dining experience.

Cafe

Solid Rock Cafe

Hours:
7am-9pm daily

Shop 30-32A, G/F,
Discovery Bay Plaza,
Discovery Bay,
Lantau Island

Takeaway: Yes
Credit Cards: V,MC

2987 1945

The Solid Rock Café looks 'country style' and generally offers jazzed-up sandwiches and some other predictable café meals. The attached bakery, however, offers some delicious breads and pastries to take away.

As an example of the café fare: gourmet grilled panini (with mixed cheese and a choice of toppings) is $35; gourmet sandwiches (including smoked salmon with cream cheese and onion) are also $35; and quiche with pasta garden salad is $38. There's also haggis, unbaked pizza and pies to take home.

Do what the locals do - grab a pastry from here and a coffee from the coffee shop nearby and sit out in the 'square' soaking up the sunshine.

Blueberry

Pub

Shop No. 8, G/F,
2 Ngan Wan Road,
Mui Wo,
Lantau Island

2984 2779

Hours:
10am-1am daily

Takeaway: Yes
Credit Cards: None

Blueberry is a sports bar, located behind the main street near the bus station and next to Wellcome.

It offers pub food. You can order roast chicken with chips and salad for $45; spaghetti bolognaise for $37; and pork chops with vegetables and chips for $48. The tasty Thai vegetable curry is $45.

The prices aren't too bad and you can watch the football while munching and drinking. There's also parking for your bike right next to the outdoor seating area.

Pub   **China Bear**

Hours: G/F, Mui Wo Centre,
10am-3am daily   Mui Wo,
                                         Lantau Island

Takeaway: Yes
Credit Cards: None   2984 7360

Located right on the waterfront with views onto
Silvermine Bay, China Bear is more a bar than a
restaurant but you can also eat here for okay
prices.

For 'Quick Bites', the tacos are not bad at $45 and
the tuna melt is $48. The steak sandwich for $50
and the veggi burger for $45 are regular China
Bear dishes. Larger, 'Mega Bite' meals are
available for $65 or more.

Seating is available inside and outside, and with a
pool table and the football on TV, this is a great
place to spend a pleasant afternoon or evening
waiting for the elusive 'next' ferry.

Fuk Chui Loi / Tak Juk Kee   Chinese

No. 1 & 3 Chung Hau Rd.,
Mui Wo,
Lantau Island

2984 8227/2984 1265

Hours:
12pm-3pm
& 6pm-10pm daily

Takeaway: Yes
Credit Cards: V,MC

These two restaurants share the same view over Silvermine Bay and have similar menu offerings and prices. Perched on a small hill, the view from the restaurants is one of the best in Mui Wo.

The seafood offered at the restaurants is quite expensive except if you go for the typically cheaper option - squid. Most non-seafood and squid dishes are around the $50 mark including squid with vegetable, squid in curry sauce and diced pork with cashew nuts.

Both restaurants are geared up to take large groups and buying in bulk would make the prices of the seafood more reasonable.

Italian   **La Pizzeria**

Hours:
10am-11pm daily

Takeaway: Yes
Credit Cards: None

2984 8933

For a small place, Mui Wo is well endowed with Italian (or Italian-sounding) restaurants and this is one example. La Pizzeria offers inside and outside seating and is located right next to The Hippo Pub (also reviewed).

The restaurant offers a range of pastas and pizzas as well as some non-Italian main dishes - for example, vegetable curry ($60) and fajitas ($78). The pizzas are all the usual types (including a Cajun chicken pizza) and come with a large amount of melted cheese, averaging from $55 for a small to $85 for a large that can easily be shared.

The pasta dishes sound quite authentic and include: penne all' pesto (which comes with shrimps) for $52 and spaghetti all' pollo for $55.

Rome Restaurant

Chinese

G/F, Ngan Fai Building,
Mui Wo Ferry Pier Road,
Lantau Island

2984 7982

Hours:
11am–10.30pm daily

Takeaway: Yes
Credit Cards: None

Don't be fooled by the name, this restaurant offers no Italian but mainly Chinese food.

Prices are very cheap here - most dishes are around $30 and there are sets available for $36 and up. Vermicelli and noodle in soup dishes range from $20, to $25 for sliced garoupa noodle in soup. As a sample of other prices and fare: fried udon with pork is $32; beef curry with rice is $28; and fried rice with mixed vegetables is $28.

The '70s decor doesn't seem to affect the restaurant's popularity with the locals, so if you feel like a Chinese meal then this is a place to visit.

Pub   **The Hippo Pub**

Hours:
M to F: 4pm-12am
Sa, Su & PH: 11am-12am

Takeaway: Yes
Credit Cards: None

G/F, Grand View
Mansion, Mui Wo Ferry
Pier Rd, Mui Wo,
Lantau Island

2984 9876

Next door and sharing the same laneway for
outside seating as La Pizzeria (also reviewed), is
The Hippo Pub.

It's a local's pub and offers regular quiz nights for
patrons. The décor is very 'pubbish' with the
standard bar and stool seats and the atmosphere
is quite cosy and friendly. There are meals
available but they don't come cheap - there's
nothing below $60 for a main meal. For example,
the Hippo burger, the lasagne, the veggie pastie
and the chilli con carne are all $60 each.

When in Rome do as the Romans do, and enjoy a
pint here after a hike or a beach visit before
heading back home.

Po Lin

Chinese

Ngong Ping,
Lantau Island

Hours:
11:30am-5pm daily

2985 5248

Takeaway: Yes
Credit Cards: None

Operated by the monks of Po Lin, there are two kinds of meals available at this well-known vegetarian restaurant - either a set vegetarian meal eaten inside at set meal times, or the snack meal that can be eaten under cover outside at any time.

For the set meal, you must buy a meal ticket before eating - either a general ticket for $60 or the deluxe ticket for $100. The general ticket price includes the admission fee to the Big Buddha as well as the set meal - not a bad deal for both 'attractions'. The tasty meal includes soup and noodles with a sample of vegetables grown locally. The snack meal will set you back $10 for a small plate of noodles with some vegetables and $10 for a selection of three yummy desserts.

If you're visiting the Big Buddha, and you like vegetarian food, then this place is worth a visit.

Indian / Italian

India to Italy

Hours:
Tu to F: 11am-3pm
& 6pm-11pm
Sa & Su: 11am-11pm
Takeaway: Yes
Credit Cards: V,MC,AE,D

40-Rear, Peng Chau
Wing On Street,
Peng Chau

2983 1188

Don't feel confused if you hear Indian music while eating your complimentary pappadums, and waiting for your lasagne to arrive.

Like the rest of the eateries here, this place packs out on Sundays with D.B. adventurers but during the week you can have the place to yourself. Technically, this restaurant shouldn't make it into this guide as most dishes are $70 or above for a main meal. But as there is a dearth of restaurants on the island, and because it's the best one in town, it's worth a mention.

The menu offers both Indian and Italian cuisine, as the name suggests, and the food is good. Menu items include tandoori specialities, such as fish or chicken tikka; and spaghetti carbonara and a range of pizzas.

Joy Inn

50 Wing On Street,
Peng Chau

Hours:
5pm-12am daily

2983 9772

Takeaway: Yes
Credit Cards: V

Peng Chau

Joy Inn is quite cute with its English-looking small picket fence and flowerpots marking a small plot in the town square area.

This place is both a bar and an eatery with small booth seats inside and the standard plastic furniture outside. The food available is Western in appeal, including: spaghetti carbonara and chilli con carne for $48; tom yum kung for $50 and regular pizzas for $50.

Don't come here for lunch because nothing gets going until later in the afternoon.

Chinese

Posture Desserts

Hours:
M to Sa: 6am–7.30pm
Su: 12pm-8pm

Shop 30, G/F, Ka Fai
Shopping Arcade,
Peng Chau

Takeaway: Yes
Credit Cards: None

2983 8182

Located near the ferry pier, this little 'hole in the wall' shop is very cheap, offering Chinese fare and some other items. You can sit behind the shopfront in the small restaurant or out on the town square with the elderly locals.

$20 can buy you a rice or noodle dish, for example, pork chop or sautéed cabbage and shredded meat. Set lunches are $28, or you can opt for a sushi roll for $10 or a hot dog for the same price. There's a bakery two doors down selling bread items to supplement your meal here if you like.

While there's nothing flash about this place, the food is among the cheapest on the island and is good for a snack if nothing else.

The Forest Bar   Thai / Western

G/F, 38C,
Wing Hing Street,
Peng Chau

Hours:
M: Closed
Tu to Su: 11am-11pm

Takeaway: Yes
Credit Cards: V,MC

2983 8837

In sync with the Peng Chau theme of cuisine combinations, this bar/restaurant offers Thai/Western food in an attempted English pub atmosphere.

If you didn't know about this place, you'd probably never find it. It's out of the 'tourist way' but it's worth a visit if you like snooker. Again, the food prices are rather expensive, especially the prawn and crab dishes, but there are some cheaper items such as: sweet and sour pork/chicken (Thai style) for $50; Thai curry for $62; deep fried pork/chicken with garlic and pepper for $42; and pad Thai for $48.

The food is not great value (in price or taste) so the snooker table is the main draw-card here.

Brief Bites

Here is some brief information on some more good-value restaurants located throughout Hong Kong:

Hong Kong Island

Central
For the best egg tart in town, according to Chris Patten, Hong Kong's last colonial governor, visit the **Tai Chong Bakery** (G/F, 32 Lyndhurst Terrace, Central, 2544 3475).

Cheap juices, including mango juice for $8 and orange juice for $5, are available at two busy juice outlets located right on the street on the corner of Wellington Street and Cochrane Street, under the Mid-Levels Escalator.

Pasta E Pizza (Basement 11, Lyndhurst Terrace, Central, 2545 1675) serves up good pizzas that are reasonably priced when shared between friends.

The **L16 Modern Thai Cuisine restaurant** (Hong Kong Park, Cotton Tree Drive, Central, 2522 6333) offers just that in a tranquil setting - in the middle of Hong Kong Park. Main meals are around $70, and seating is offered both inside and out.

TW Café (No. 2, G/F, Capitol Plaza, 2-10 Lyndhurst Terrace, Central, 2544 2237) is a coffee specialist and is a nice place to enjoy some morning or afternoon tea.

They sell different kinds of freshly brewed coffee, tea, and food and snacks.

The Globe (39 Hollywood Road, Central, 2543 1941) is a pub but it does offer meals - including the delicious avocado chicken melt - for decent prices. Plus it's open from 7.30am in the mornings (Monday to Friday) if you want an early morning fry-up.

Happy Valley
At **Liz's Cheesecake shop** (G/F, No. 69E, Sing Woo Road, Happy Valley, 2893 3394) you can enjoy a pleasant afternoon tea outing with cheesecake for $23 per piece, or coffee and cake deals from $35. Whole cheesecakes are also available.

Pizzeria Italia (77 Sing Woo Road, Happy Valley, 2572 5710 and 17-19 Mosque Street, Mid-Levels, 2525 2519) has pizzas that work out to be reasonably priced when shared (for example, the Salami Piccante - margherita with spicy salami - is $110). All pizzas come with a complimentary litre bottle of Lissa Mineral Water.

Tai Hong Street, Sai Wan Ho
Dubbed as 'SOHO East', a few restaurants have sprung up along Tai Hong Street in Sai Wan Ho. With harbour views over to Kowloon, the following restaurants are worth checking out if you are in the area. **Eastern Coast** (Shop GA10A, G/F, 55 Tai Hong Street, Lei King Wan, Sai Wan Ho, 2977 5422) is popular and offers casual, open-air, Chinese style dining with everything $30 or less. **Chit Chat Restaurant and Bar** (GA8-9, Kwung Fung Mansion, Lei King Wan, Sai Wan Ho, 2967 1666) is part of a chain along the street and offers a fine dining atmosphere with sets around $60, and

Chinese and Western style mains from $30. **Beira Rio**
(Shop GB08-10, G/F, 45 Tai Hong Street, Lei King Wan,
Sai Wan Ho, 2568 3993) also offers fine dining; for
example, baked lamb chop with garlic or mushroom,
and tea or coffee, for $48.

Wanchai
For one of the best views in town, in air-conditioned
comfort and with a range of restaurants to choose
from, the **Hong Kong Convention and Exhibition
Centre** (1 Expo Drive, Wanchai, 2582 8888) is worth a
visit. For eating with a view and budget in mind, check
out: the **Port Café**, which has main Western style
meals at around $70 each; the **Cyber Café** which
offers snacks including desserts and drinks for around
$20 each (along with free Internet access for diners);
and the **Harbour Lounge**, which caters more for
buffet diners.

Deluxe Sandwiches Express (9 Luard Road,
Wanchai, 2527 1328) is a cheap place to get a
sandwich. For example, European style sandwich sets
(sandwich and drink) are $20 while Hong Kong style
sandwich sets are $15.

Sun Channel (G/F, MLC Tower, 248 Queens Road East,
Wanchai, 2285 8388) also offers Western style fare,
including pasta for around $50 and lemon cheesecake
for $22.

In general, there are many, many restaurants to
choose from in Wanchai, particularly inside the square
bound by **O'Brien Road, Hennessy Road, Fenwick
Street** and **Jaffe Road**, where you'll find plenty of
cheap options, not only local style, that are open all
day and well into the night too.

Kowloon

Jordan
Nachghar Himalayan Cultural Club (54 Jordan Road, Jordan, 2311 1415) is largely frequented by Nepalese expatriates which is a good sign of its authenticity and cheapness.

Kowloon City
Where there are Thai restaurants, there always seems to be good food. Kowloon City is no exception.
Golden Orchard Thai Restaurant (12 Lung Kong Road, Kowloon City, 2383 3076) is popular, albeit a bit smoky. Look for the well-kept shrine out the front.

Lanna Thai Restaurant (G/F, 15 Tak Ku Ling Road, Kowloon City, 2718 2201) offers good value set lunches (including rice, main meal, dessert and a drink) between 11.30am and 3pm for $25 or $35.

If you are looking for a different cuisine type, **the Indian Restaurant** (G/F, 24 South Wall Road, Kowloon City, 2716 5128) offers an economical taste of India with a lunch set for $38.

New Territories

Sai Kung
The alleyways in the old town of **Sai Kung**, just near the bus terminal, are teeming with cheap eateries. The food is mostly Chinese style with most dishes on offer for $25 or less.

Tuen Mun/Sham Tseng

If you're feeling spiritual (and hungry), the monks and helpers at the **Miu Fat Buddhist Monastery** (18 Castle Peak Road, Lam Tei, Tuen Mun, 2461 8567) cook up a healthy and filling vegetarian lunch feast for $75 each (or $70 per head if you have ten people or more).

The village of Sham Tseng is famous for its goose restaurants. The **Nang Kee Roast Goose Restaurant** (Sham Tseng Sun Tsuen, Sham Tseng, 2491 0392) is worth a try; the average price for a dish is $50 and one whole roasted goose is $230 (which can easily be shared by up to ten people).

Outlying Islands

Cheung Chau

Some 'snackeries' open only on a seasonal basis - 7 days a week during the swimming months but only on the weekends in winter. One of them is **Hoi Bun**, located at the entrance to Tung Wan beach (1 Tung Wan Road, 2981 8216). This place also offers prospective barbecue enthusiasts all the necessary BBQ items (forks, charcoal and food) at reasonable prices.

Opposite Hoi Bun, **Pok Oi** (same address and phone number) transforms itself into a bar, serving alcoholic drinks in the evening, that is popular with weekenders and locals alike.

Further along the beach, and with fine views over Tung Wan Beach and Afternoon Beach, is the **Windsurfing and Water Sports Centre** (1 Hak Pai Road, Kwun Yam Wan, 2981 8316). It's a great place to relax and watch windsurfers ply the calm waters.

Lamma Island

Seafood restaurants abound on Lamma, and eating at them is more economical if you dine with a large group. In Yung Shue Wan, the **Lamma Seaview and Man Fung Seafood Restaurant** (No. 5 Main Street, 2982 0719) offers 184 menu items. Its specialities are fried lobster with cheese and fried prawn with garlic butter. **The Sampan Seafood Restaurant** (16 Main Street, 2982 2388) offers standard market-priced seafood with prices for seafood dishes starting at $65.

In Sok Kwu Wan, the **Rainbow Seafood Restaurant** (1A-1B, 23-24 & 16-20 First Street, 2982 8100) is huge with three 'outlets' and provides free ferry transport for diners. The **Tai Yuen Restaurant** (15 First Street, 2982 8386) is probably the cheapest of the restaurants in this part of Lamma. For example, calamari dishes are offered at $42.

Lantau Island

If you're feeling like some really tasty Italian with a nice beach view, **Brezza** (G/F, D.B. Plaza, Discovery Bay, 2914 1906) is the place to go. The prices are not cheap though, with everything over $70. So if you're on a budget, your best option is to share one of the mouth-watering pizzas (average $80).

Quick Reference Guide

By Location

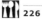

Non-Smoking Section

Vegetarian

Lamma Island

Lantau Island

Tsim Sha Tsui

Wanchai

Branches

Blue Bird	Japanese
Lamma Island	2982 0687
Ap Lei Chau	2518 3683

Café Very Good	Chinese
Central	2545 9005
Happy Valley	2838 3318

Chilli n' Spice	Asian
Stanley	2899 0147
Causeway Bay	2504 3930
Lantau Island	2987 9191
Sha Tin	2693 3128
Tsim Sha Tsui	2312 1118

CitySuper	Food Hall
Causeway Bay	2506 2888
Tsim Sha Tsui	2272 0812

Dailybread Café	Café
Central, LKF	2868 6013
Central	2259 9088
Central, IFC	2295 3889

Ebeneezer's	International
Lantau Island	2987 0036
Wanchai	2529 3738

Jo Jo Indian	Indian
Lantau Island	2987 0122
Tsuen Wan	2416 5553

Jo Jo Mess Club	Indian
Causeway Bay	2894 9722
Central	2522 6209
Wanchai	2527 3776

King's Palace	Chinese
Happy Valley	2838 4444
Kowloon Tong	2265 7777

Kung Tak Lam	Shanghainese
Tsim Sha Tsui	2367 7881
Causeway Bay	2890 3127

Macau	Macanese
Tsim Sha Tsui	2366 8148
Tsim Sha Tsui	2721 0219
Tsim Sha Tsui	2301 1999

Mak's Noodles	Chinese
Central	2854 3810
Causeway Bay	2895 5310

Pizza Milano	Italian
Lamma Island	2982 4848
Central	2581 2848

Mini Paris	Vietnamese
Causeway Bay	2591 4015
Tsuen Wan	2415 1573
Sha Tin	2604 8336

Mix	Cafe
Central, IFC	2971 0688
Central	2523 7396
Quarry Bay	2562 7313

Moon House	Chinese
Causeway Bay	2882 3737
Happy Valley	2891 2591

Nine to Five	International
Central	2840 1073
Central, IFC	2295 0100

Pho Saigon	Vietnamese
Mongkok	2142 7747
Wanchai	2833 6833

Pret A Manger	Cafe
Causeway Bay	2808 4230
Central, IFC	2520 0445
Central	2537 9230

Taiwan Chicken	Taiwanese
Kowloon City	2926 6018
Tsim Sha Tsui	2926 3088

Tiffany	International
Mongkok	2381 1516
Wanchai	2836 3381

Notes

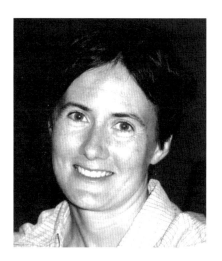

About the Author
Hailing from gastronomical Melbourne and married to a career foodie, Nicole Lade was eager to explore the Hong Kong food scene when she arrived in the SAR in June, 2001.

A terrible cook and suddenly unemployed in the tech crash, Nicole found herself eating out a lot and actively searching for cheap but good value restaurants.

The results of her quest led to monthly restaurant review contributions to the Hong Kong Town Crier magazine and now to this new and useful first-of-its-kind guide.